Bone Marrow Transplants

A Book of Basics for Patients

by

Susan K. Stewart

Medical Editors:

Martin S. Tallman MD   *Patrick J. Stiff MD*

Bone Marrow Transplants:
A Book of Basics for Patients

Published by:
BMT Newsletter
1985 Spruce Ave.
Highland Park, Illinois 60035
708-831-1913

ISBN 0-9647352-0-2

Publication of this book made possible in part by a grant from:

Immunex Corporation

Special thanks to:
Desktop Edit Shop, Skokie, Illinois, design and typesetting
Cheryl Steiger, cover design and illustrations
Richard Hong, MD, illustrations

ACKNOWLEDGMENTS

Special thanks to the following physicians, nurses and psychiatric counselors who served as medical advisors for the first twelve issues of BMT Newsletter that form the basis of this book, and without whose help this book would not be possible:

Tauseef Ahmed MD
New York Medical College,
    Valhalla NY

Linda D. Applegarth ED.D
Center for Reproductive
    Medicine and Infertility
Cornell University Medical
    College, New York City NY

Patrick Beatty MD PhD
University of Utah Medical
    School, Salt Lake City UT

Richard E. Champlin MD
MD Anderson Cancer Center,
    Houston TX

Roberta Dillon RN MSN
University of Virginia Health
    Sciences Center, Charlottesville
    VA

Robert Geller MD
Emory University School of
    Medicine, Atlanta GA

John Graham-Pole MD MRCP
University of Florida College of
    Medicine, Gainesville FL

Richard Hong MD
University of Wisconsin
    Hospitals, Madison WI

Herbert Kaizer MD
Rush Presbyterian St. Luke's
    Medical Center, Chicago IL

Anne Kessinger MD
University of Nebraska Medical
    Center, Omaha NE

Morris Kletzel MD
Children's Memorial Hospital,
    Chicago IL

Mary Lauer RN PNP
Children's Hospital of Wisconsin,
    Milwaukee WI

Irving Leon PhD
University of Michigan, Ann
    Arbor MI

George B. McDonald MD
Fred Hutchinson Cancer
    Research Center, Seattle WA

Philip McGlave MD
University of Minnesota Hospital
    & Clinics, Minneapolis MN

Daniel Pietryga MD
Children's Hospital of Wisconsin,
    Milwaukee WI

Debbie Richards RN BSN
Children's Hospital of Wisconsin,
    Milwaukee WI

Jean Sanders MD
Fred Hutchinson Cancer
    Research Center, Seattle WA

Mark V. Sauer MD
California Reproductive Health
    Institute
University of Southern California,
    Los Angeles CA

Richard L. Schilsky MD
University of Chicago Pritzker
    School of Medicine, Chicago IL

Patrick J. Stiff MD
Loyola University Medical
    Center, Maywood IL

Aimee St. Pierre MD
Rush Presbyterian St. Luke's
    Medical Center, Chicago IL

Martin S. Tallman MD
Northwestern University Medical
    School, Chicago IL

Georgia Vogelsang MD
Johns Hopkins Oncology Center,
    Baltimore MD

Stephanie Williams MD
University of Chicago Pritzker
    School of Medicine, Chicago IL

Jane Winter MD
Northwestern University Medical
    School, Chicago IL

Thanks also to the following BMT patients, family members and other technical advisors whose experiences and expertise are shared in this book:

Cindy Barkdull PhD.
Nancy Beskin
Lorraine Boldt
Georgia Comfort
Thelda D.
Sue and Steve Freeman
Ann Glowinski
Connie Hannes
Judith Kaufman
Ruth Krueger
Susan Mitchell
Gail P.
Jerry Schwartz
Mary Scherer

Pat Tabet
Caesar Tabet
Michelle Vandermaas
Ellyn Weiselman
Ted Wieseman
Jacqueline Williams
Janet Winkowski
Laura Wise

And especially to Thomas Stewart and Mary Ann Chandler, who've been invaluable sources of help and encouragement in producing BMT Newsletter.

Dear Friend,

In 1988, after being diagnosed with leukemia, my doctor recommended a bone marrow transplant. I'd never before heard of a bone marrow transplant, and hadn't a clue as to what bone marrow is or why it's important.

I was confused and overwhelmed. All the medical terms used to describe a BMT were new to me, and often I was so lost I couldn't even figure out the right questions to ask! After recovering from my BMT, I met several other BMT survivors and learned my experience was not unique.

This book is written *by* patients *for* patients with the help of several doctors and nurses. It's designed to "translate" some of the medical information you'll receive before, during and after your bone marrow transplant into plain English.

There's no getting around it—bone marrow transplantation is a big, confusing subject. There's lots of information to absorb in this book. Take it at your own pace.

If you're only ready for the basics, start with Chapters 1 and 6. Then use the table of contents and index to find answers to the questions that are bothering you most.

When you're ready, read the other chapters for a more in-depth explanation of the different kinds of transplants, complications that can arise, and how other patients have coped with the experience.

I know how difficult it is to make the decision to have a bone marrow transplant, undergo the treatment, and get back to a normal life. I hope this book helps make your experience a little easier.

Susan Stewart

Susan K. Stewart
Editor, BMT Newsletter

P.S. The first 12 issues of the BMT Newsletter form the basis of this book. BMT Newsletter is a free publication for BMT patients, survivors and their families. If you'd like your name added to the circulation list, call 708-831-1913.

TABLE OF CONTENTS

1. The Nuts and Bolts of Bone Marrow Transplants 11
    What is Bone Marrow? 11
    Why a Transplant? 11
    Types of Transplant...12
    Preparing for the Transplant..13
    Bone Marrow Harvest 13
        Ill. 1 Bone marrow harvest 13
    Preparative Regimen 14
        Ill. 2 Hickman catheter 14
    The Transplant 15
    Engraftment 15
    What a Patient Feels During the Transplant.................................16
    Handling Emotional Stress 17
    Leaving the Hospital..18
    Life after Transplant...18
    Is It Worth It? 19

2. Some Fundamentals about Blood Cells....................................21
    Blood Cell Production..22
        Ill. 1 How blood cells develop 22

3. Autologous Bone Marrow Transplants 25
    Who Is a Candidate for an Autologous BMT? 25
        Hodgkin's and Non-Hodgkin's Lymphomas 26
        Leukemia..27
        Breast Cancer 28
        Childhood Neuroblastoma 29
        Other Diseases..30
    Purging Bone Marrow 30
    Post-Recovery 31
    Georgia Comfort...31

4. Allogeneic Bone Marrow Transplants 33
        Fig. 1 Diseases Frequently Treated with Allogeneic BMTs 33
    The HLA System 34
        Ill. 1 Allogeneic BMTs 34
        Ill. 2 Antigen matches..35
        Fig. 2 Inheritance of HLA-Antigens 36
        HLA-Matching 37
        HLA-Typing Test...37
    Matched Related Donors...38
        Acute Myelogenous Leukemia (AML)......................................38

Acute Lymphocytic Leukemia (ALL) 39
Chronic Myelogenous Leukemia (CML) 39
Hodgkin's and Non-Hodgkin's Lymphomas 39
Aplastic Anemia 40
Mis-Matched BMTS **40**
Unrelated Donor Transplants **41**
Searching for an Unrelated Donor **42**
Being a Donor **43**
Laura Wise **44**

5. PERIPHERAL STEM CELL TRANSPLANTS **47**
Stem Cells **47**
Peripheral Stem Cell Harvest **48**
Fig. 1 Diseases Treated with PSC Transplants 48
Ill. 1 Peripheral stem cell harvest 49
Reasons for PSCHS **49**
Pros and Cons of PSCHS **49**
Thelda D. **50**

6. EMOTIONAL AND PSYCHOLOGICAL CONSIDERATIONS **53**
Coping with the News **53**
Getting Information **54**
Setting Goals **54**
Ill. 1 Congratulations 55
Loss of Control **55**
Fig. 1 Tips for Patients 56
Isolation **57**
Physical Discomfort **58**
Psychiatric Help **59**
Being There for the Patient **59**
Ill. 2 Talk with a counselor 60
Getting Back to Normal **61**
Fig. 2 Tips for Support Persons 62
And Many Months Beyond **63**
Poem: Unready Heroes **64**

7. WHEN YOUR CHILD NEEDS A BONE MARROW TRANSPLANT **67**
Deciding on a BMT **67**
Getting Information **68**
Preparing for the Transplant **70**
Ill. 1 Visiting the hospital before admission 72
Siblings' Concerns **72**
The Sibling Donor **73**
Waiting for the Transplant **73**

Life During Transplant 74
    Ill. 2 Make the hospital room your own 75
Going Home 77

8. INFECTIONS 81
Fighting Infection—The Immune System 82
    Lymphocytes...82
    Other Leukocytes 83
Bacterial Infections 83
Fungal Infections...85
    Fig. 1 Usual Causes of Infection Post-Transplant 85
Viral Infections..86
    Herpes Simplex 86
    Cytomegalovirus..87
    Varicella Zoster Virus 88
    Other Viruses 88
    Fig. 2 Preventing Infections..................................89
Protozoa 90
Don't Take Chances 90

9. GRAFT-VERSUS-HOST DISEASE...91
T-cells...91
GVHD 92
Acute GVHD 92
    Fig. 1 Stages of Acute GVHD 93
    Prevention & Treatment of Acute GVHD 93
    T-cell Depletion 94
Chronic GVHD 95
    Treatment of Chronic GVHD.................................96
    Fig. 2 Symptoms/Side Effects of Chronic GVHD 96
Long-Term Concerns..97
Coping with the Stress of GVHD 97
Susan Mitchell 99

10. LIVER COMPLICATIONS..101
    Fig. 1 Signs of Liver Problems 102
During the First Three Months after a BMT 102
    Veno-Occlusive Disease..102
    Acute GVHD of the Liver 104
    Bloodstream Infections 104
    Fungal Liver Disease...104
    Drug-Induced Liver Injury 105
    Viral Hepatitis...106
    Biliary Disease 106

After the Third Month Post-Transplant..106
    Chronic GVHD of the Liver..107
    Chronic Viral Hepatitis..107
    Fungal Liver Disease...107

11. INFERTILITY **109**
  Steps to Pregnancy **110**
    Ill. 1 Reproductive organs 110
  Sperm Production..**111**
  Chemotherapy & Radiation..**112**
    Fig. 1 Drugs that Can Cause Infertility 113
  Medically Assisted Reproduction................................**114**
    Artificial Insemination 114
    In-vitro Fertilization 116
    Choosing a Program...118
    Emotional Considerations..119
  The Adoption Option..**119**
    Agency-Assisted Adoption..119
    Private Adoption 120
    Cost...121
    Emotional Considerations 121

12. INSURANCE AND BONE MARROW TRANSPLANTS............**123**
  What Types of Insurance Are Available? **124**
    Private Insurance 124
    Self-Insured...125
    HMOs (Health Maintenance Organizations)..............125
    Government Programs...126
    Other Plans 126
    Fig. 1 Comprehensive Health Insurance Plans......................127
    Fig. 2 Blue Cross/Blue Shield Open Enrollment................128
  Is Your Health Insurance Adequate?...........................**127**
  When Insurance Says No… **128**
    What's the Problem? 129
    Experimental/Investigative 129
    Not Medically Necessary...130
    Not Eligible...131
    Usual and Customary...131
    Fig. 3 Don't Take No for an Answer 132
    Going to Court 133
  BMT Newsletter 1991 Insurance Survey **133**
  Gail P. **134**

APPENDIX A: UNDERSTANDING BLOOD TESTS............................**137**

APPENDIX B: RESOURCES 141

APPENDIX C: GLOSSARY OF TERMS...151

INDEX..159

CHAPTER 1

The Nuts and Bolts of Bone Marrow Transplants

Bone marrow transplantation (BMT) is a relatively new medical procedure being used to treat diseases once thought incurable. Since its first successful use in 1968, BMTs have been used to treat patients diagnosed with leukemia, aplastic anemia, lymphomas such as Hodgkin's disease, multiple myeloma, immune deficiency disorders and some solid tumors such as breast and ovarian cancer.

In 1991, more than 7,500 people underwent BMTs nationwide. Although BMTs now save thousands of lives each year, 70 percent of those needing a BMT using donor marrow are unable to have one because a suitable bone marrow donor cannot be found.

WHAT IS BONE MARROW?

Bone marrow is a spongy tissue found inside bones. The bone marrow in the breast bone, skull, hips, ribs and spine contains stem cells that produce the body's blood cells. These blood cells include white blood cells (leukocytes), which fight infection; red blood cells (erythrocytes), which carry oxygen to and remove waste products from organs and tissues; and platelets, which enable the blood to clot.

WHY A TRANSPLANT?

In patients with leukemia, aplastic anemia, and some immune deficiency diseases, the stem cells in the bone marrow malfunction, producing an excessive number of defective or immature blood cells (in the case of leukemia) or low blood cell counts (in the case of aplastic anemia). The immature or defective blood cells interfere with the production of normal blood cells, accumulate in the bloodstream and may invade other tissues.

Large doses of chemotherapy and/or radiation are required to destroy the abnormal stem cells and abnormal blood cells. These therapies, however, not only kill the abnormal cells but can destroy normal cells found in the bone marrow as well. Similarly, aggressive chemotherapy used to treat some lymphomas and other cancers can destroy healthy bone marrow. A bone marrow transplant enables physicians to treat these diseases with aggressive chemotherapy and/or radiation by allowing replacement of the diseased or damaged bone marrow after the chemotherapy/radiation treatment.

While bone marrow transplants do not provide 100 percent assurance that the disease will not recur, a transplant can increase the likelihood of a cure or at least prolong the period of disease-free survival for many patients.

TYPES OF TRANSPLANT

In a bone marrow transplant, the patient's diseased bone marrow is destroyed and healthy marrow is infused into the patient's bloodstream. In a successful transplant, the new bone marrow migrates to the cavities of the large bones, engrafts and begins producing normal blood cells.

If bone marrow from a donor is used, the transplant is called an "allogeneic" BMT, or "syngeneic" BMT if the donor is an identical twin. In an allogeneic BMT, the new bone marrow infused into the patient must match the genetic makeup of the patient's own marrow as perfectly as possible. Special blood tests are conducted to determine whether or not the donor's bone marrow matches the patient's. If the donor's bone marrow is not a good genetic match, it will perceive the patient's body as foreign material to be attacked and destroyed. This condition is known as graft-versus-host disease (GVHD) and can be life-threatening. Alternatively, the patient's immune system may destroy the new bone marrow. This is called graft rejection.

There is a 35 percent chance that a patient will have a sibling whose bone marrow is a perfect match. If the patient has no matched sibling, a donor may be located in one of the international bone marrow donor registries, or a mis-matched or autologous transplant may be considered.

In some cases, patients may be their own bone marrow donors. This is called an autologous BMT and is possible if the disease afflicting the bone marrow is in remission or if the condition being treated does not involve the bone marrow (e.g. breast cancer, ovarian cancer, Hodgkin's

Disease, non-Hodgkin's lymphoma, and brain tumors). The bone marrow is extracted from the patient prior to transplant and may be "purged" to remove lingering malignant cells (if the disease has afflicted the bone marrow).

PREPARING FOR THE TRANSPLANT

A successful transplant requires the patient be healthy enough to undergo the rigors of the transplant procedure. Age, general physical condition, the patient's diagnosis and the stage of the disease are all considered by the physician when determining whether a person should undergo a transplant.

Prior to a bone marrow transplant, a battery of tests is carried out to ensure the patient is physically capable of undergoing a transplant. Tests of the patient's heart, lung, kidney and other vital organ functions are also used to develop a patient "baseline" against which post-transplant tests can be compared to determine if any body functions have been impaired. The pre-transplant tests are usually done on an outpatient basis.

A successful bone marrow transplant requires an expert medical team—doctors, nurses, and other support staff—who are experienced in bone marrow transplants, can promptly recognize problems and emerging side effects, and know how to react swiftly and properly if problems do arise. A good bone marrow transplant program will also recognize the importance of providing patients and their families with emotional and psychological support before, during and after the transplant, and will make personnel and other support systems readily available to families for this purpose.

BONE MARROW HARVEST

Regardless of whether the patient or a donor provides the bone marrow used in the transplant, the procedure used to collect the marrow— the bone marrow harvest—is the same. The bone marrow harvest takes place in a hospital operating room, usually under general anesthesia. It involves little risk and minimal discomfort.

While the patient is under anesthesia, a needle is inserted into the cavity of the rear hip bone or "iliac crest" where a large quantity of bone marrow is located. The bone marrow—a thick, red liquid—is extracted with a needle and syringe. Several skin punctures on each hip and multiple bone punctures are usually required to extract the requisite amount of bone marrow. There are no surgical incisions or stitches involved—only skin punctures where the needle was inserted.

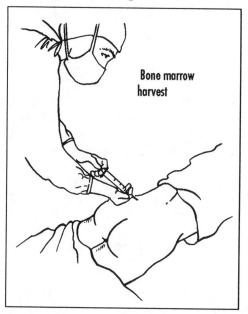

Bone marrow harvest

The amount of bone marrow harvested depends on the size of the patient and the concentration of bone marrow cells in the donor's blood. Usually one to two quarts of marrow and blood are harvested. While this may sound like a lot, it really only represents about 2% of a person's bone marrow, which the body replaces in four weeks.

When the anesthesia wears off, the donor may feel some discomfort at the harvest site. The pain will be similar to that associated with a hard fall on the ice and can usually be controlled with Tylenol. Donors who are not also the BMT patient are usually discharged after an overnight stay and can fully resume normal activities in a few days.

For autologous transplants, the harvested bone marrow will be frozen (cryopreserved) and stored at a temperature between -80 and -196 degrees centigrade until the day of transplant. It may first be "purged" to remove residual cancerous cells that can't be easily identified under the microscope (see page 30).

In allogeneic BMTs, the bone marrow may be treated to remove "T-cells" (T-cell depletion) to reduce the risk of graft-versus-host disease (see page 94). It will then be transferred directly to the patient's room for infusion.

PREPARATIVE REGIMEN

A patient admitted to the bone marrow transplant unit will first undergo several days of chemotherapy and/or radiation which destroys bone marrow and cancerous cells and makes room for the new bone marrow. This is called the conditioning or preparative regimen.

The exact regimen of chemotherapy and/or radiation varies according to the disease being treated and the "protocol" or preferred treatment plan of the facility where the BMT is being performed.

Prior to conditioning, a small flexible tube called a catheter (sometimes called a "Hickman" or central venous line) will be inserted into a large vein in the patient's chest just above the heart. This tube enables the medical staff to administer drugs and blood products to the patient painlessly, and to withdraw the hundreds of blood samples required during the course of treatment without inserting needles into the patient's arms or hands.

The dosage of chemotherapy and/or radiation given to patients during conditioning is much stronger than dosages administered to patients with the same disease who are not undergoing a BMT. Patients may become weak, irritable and nauseated. Most BMT centers administer anti-nausea medications to minimize discomfort.

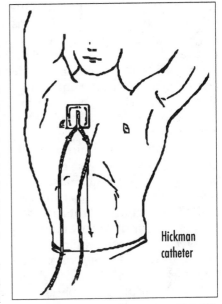

Hickman catheter

THE TRANSPLANT

A day or two following the chemotherapy and/or radiation treatment, the transplant will occur. The bone marrow is infused into the patient intravenously in much the same way that any blood product is given. The transplant is not a surgical procedure. It takes place in the patient's room, not an operating room.

Patients are checked frequently for signs of fever, chills, hives and chest pains while the bone marrow is being infused. When the transplant is completed, the days and weeks of waiting begin.

ENGRAFTMENT

The two to four weeks immediately following transplant are the most critical. The high-dose chemotherapy and/or radiation given to the patient during conditioning will have destroyed the patient's bone marrow, crippling the body's "immune" or defense system. As the patient waits for the transplanted bone marrow to migrate to the cavities of the large bones, set up housekeeping or "engraft," and begin producing normal blood cells, he or she will be very susceptible to infection and excessive bleeding. Multiple antibiotics and blood transfusions will be administered to the patient to help prevent and fight infection. Transfusions of platelets will be given to prevent bleeding. Allogeneic patients will receive additional medications to prevent and control graft-versus-host disease.

Extraordinary precautions will be taken to minimize the patient's exposure to viruses and bacteria. Visitors and hospital personnel will wash their hands with antiseptic soap and, in some cases, wear protective gowns, gloves and/or masks while in the patient's room. Fresh fruits, vegetables, plants and cut flowers will be prohibited in the patient's room since they often carry fungi and bacteria that pose a risk of infection. When leaving the room, the patient may wear a mask, gown and gloves as a barrier against bacteria and virus, and as a reminder to others that he or she is susceptible to infection.

Blood samples will be taken daily to determine whether or not engraftment has occurred and to monitor organ function. When the transplanted bone marrow finally engrafts and begins producing normal blood cells, the patient will gradually be taken off the antibiotics, and blood and platelet transfusions will generally no longer be required. Once the bone marrow is producing a sufficient number of healthy red blood cells, white blood cells and platelets, the patient will be discharged from the hospital, provided no other complications have developed. BMT patients typically spend four to eight weeks in the hospital.

WHAT A PATIENT FEELS DURING THE TRANSPLANT

A bone marrow transplant is a physically, emotionally, and psychologically taxing procedure for both the patient and family. A patient needs and should seek as much help as possible to cope with the experience. "Toughing it out" on your own is not the smartest way to cope with the transplant experience.

The bone marrow transplant is a debilitating experience. Imagine the symptoms of a severe case of the flu—nausea, vomiting, fever, diarrhea, extreme weakness. Now imagine what it's like to cope with the symptoms not just for several days, but for several weeks. That approximates what a BMT patient experiences during hospitalization.

During this period the patient will feel very sick and weak. Walking, sitting up in bed for long periods of time, reading books, talking on the phone, visiting with friends or even watching TV may require more energy than the patient has to spare.

Complications can develop after a bone marrow transplant such as infection, bleeding, graft-versus-host disease, or liver disease, which can create additional discomfort. The pain, however, is usually controllable by medication. In addition, mouth sores can develop that make eating and swallowing uncomfortable. Temporary mental confusion sometimes occurs and can be quite frightening for the patient who may not realize it's only temporary. The medical staff will help the patient deal with these problems.

HANDLING EMOTIONAL STRESS

In addition to the physical discomfort associated with the transplant experience there is emotional and psychological discomfort as well. Some patients find the emotional and psychological stress more problematic than the physical discomfort.

The psychological and emotional stress stems from several factors. First, patients undergoing transplants are already traumatized by the news that they have a life-threatening disease. While the transplant offers hope for their recovery, the prospect of undergoing a long, arduous medical procedure is still not pleasant and there's no guarantee of success.

Second, patients undergoing a transplant can feel quite isolated. The special precautions taken to guard against infection while the immune system is impaired can leave a patient feeling detached from the rest of the world and cut off from normal human contact. The patient is housed in a private room, sometimes with special air-filtering equipment to purify the air. The number of visitors is restricted and visitors are asked to wear gloves, masks and/or other protective clothing to inhibit the spread of bacteria and virus while visiting the patient. When the patient leaves the room, he or she may be required to wear a protective mask, gown and/or gloves as a barrier against infection. This feeling of isolation comes at the very time in a patient's life when familiar surroundings and close physical contact with family and friends are most needed.

"Helplessness" is also a common feeling among bone marrow transplant patients, which can breed further feelings of anger or resentment. For many, it's unnerving to be totally dependent on strangers for survival, no matter how competent they may be. The fact that most patients are unfamiliar with the medical jargon used to describe the transplant procedure compounds the feeling of helplessness. Some also find it embarrassing to be dependent on strangers for help with basic daily functions such as using the washroom.

The long weeks of waiting for the transplanted marrow to engraft, for blood counts to return to safe levels, and for side effects to disappear increase the emotional trauma. Recovery can be like a roller coaster ride: one day a patient may feel much better, only to awake the next day feeling as sick as ever.

LEAVING THE HOSPITAL

After being discharged from the hospital, a patient continues recovery at home (or at lodging near the transplant center if the patient is from out of town) for two to four months. Patients usually cannot return to full-time work for up to six months after the transplant.

Though patients will be well enough to leave the hospital, their recovery will be far from over. For the first several weeks the patient may be too weak to do much more than sleep, sit up, and walk a bit around the house. Frequent visits to the hospital or associated clinic will be required to monitor the patient's progress, and to administer any medications and/or blood products needed. It can take six months or more from the day of transplant before a patient is ready to fully resume normal activities.

During this period, the patient's white blood cell counts are often too low to provide normal protection against the viruses and bacteria encountered in everyday life. Contact with the general public is therefore restricted. Crowded movie theatres, grocery stores, department stores, etc. are places recovering BMT patients avoid during their recuperation. Often patients will wear protective masks when venturing outside the home.

A patient will return to the hospital or clinic as an outpatient several times a week for monitoring, blood transfusions, and administration of other drugs as needed. Eventually, the patient becomes strong enough to resume a normal routine and to look forward to a productive, healthy life.

LIFE AFTER TRANSPLANT

It can take as long as a year for the new bone marrow to function normally. Patients are closely monitored during this time to identify any infections or complications that may develop.

Life after transplant can be both exhilarating and worrisome. On the one hand, it's exciting to be alive after being so close to death. Most patients find their quality of life improved after transplant.

Nonetheless, there is always the worry that relapse will occur. Furthermore, innocent statements or events can sometimes conjure up unpleasant memories of the transplant experience long after the patient has recovered. It can take a long time for the patient to come to grips with these difficulties.

IS IT WORTH IT?

Yes! For most patients contemplating a bone marrow transplant, the alternative is near-certain death. Despite the fact that the transplant can be a trying experience, most find that the pleasure that comes from being alive and healthy after the transplant is well worth the effort.

CHAPTER 2

Some Fundamentals about Blood Cells

Blood is composed of many different kinds of cells, each with a specific function. Most blood cells are formed in the bone marrow and released into the bloodstream at various stages of maturity.

Red blood cells (erythrocytes) make up 45 percent of blood volume. Their primary function is to pick up oxygen in the lungs and transport it to tissues throughout the body. At the tissue site, red blood cells exchange oxygen for carbon dioxide and carry it back to the lungs to be exhaled.

White blood cells (leukocytes) are only 1/1,000 as numerous as red blood cells in the bloodstream. There are five main types: neutrophils (also called granulocytes), eosinophils, basophils, monocytes, and lymphocytes. Each plays a distinct and important role in helping the immune system fight infection.

Neutrophils contain granules of bacteria-killing enzymes in the cytoplasm—the substance surrounding the cell. Eosinophils attack protozoa that cause infection. Basophils are the least common type of white blood cell and their function is not completely understood. They play an important role in regulating allergic reactions such as asthma, hives, hay fever and reactions to drugs.

Monocytes are the largest white blood cells. They engulf and destroy invading bacteria and fungi and clean up debris once foreign organisms have been destroyed by other white blood cells. When monocytes leave the bloodstream and enter tissues or organs, they can evolve into larger cells called macrophages that have an increased capacity to destroy foreign organisms invading the body.

Lymphocytes are the smallest white blood cells and are the backbone of the immune system. Lymphocytes fight viral infections and assist in the destruction of other parasites, bacteria and fungi. One group of lymphocytes called T-cells regulates the immune system's response to invading organisms and is the body's main defense against viruses and protozoa. A second group called B-cells manufactures a kind of protein called an antibody or immunoglobulin. Antibodies attach to the surface

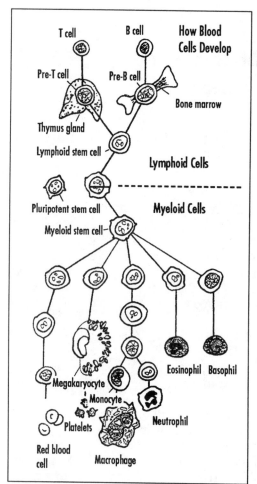

How Blood Cells Develop

of foreign organisms or the cells they have invaded and summon a group of proteins in the bloodstream called the complement system to surround the infected organism or cell and dissolve a hole in it.

Thrombocytes (platelets) are the smallest cell elements in the bloodstream. Platelets are needed to control bleeding.

BLOOD CELL PRODUCTION

New blood cells are constantly produced by the body. In healthy adults, an estimated 100 billion red cells and 400 million white cells are produced each hour. The life span of mature blood cells is short—only a few days or months.

Ninety-five percent of the body's blood cell production is believed to take place in the bone marrow. The remainder occurs in the spleen. While most blood cells produced in the bone marrow are discharged directly into the bloodstream, T-cells first travel to the thymus gland (thus, the name T-cells) where they receive further education or programming before being released into the bloodstream.

All mature blood cells are believed to originate from very primitive cells in the bone marrow called "pluripotent stem cells." This cell is capable of producing other cells identical to itself. Pluripotent stem cells also produce other stem cells—the lymphoid stem cell and the myeloid stem cell—from which the various types of mature blood cells evolve.

Like pluripotent stem cells, the myeloid and lymphoid stem cells can self-renew as well as produce colonies of offspring that eventually evolve into mature cells. However, their ability to self-renew is believed to be more limited than that of pluripotent stem cells and they are capable of producing fewer different types of offspring. Lymphoid stem cells only produce cells that evolve into lymphocytes (T-cells or B-cells). The offspring of myeloid stem cells can only evolve into either red blood cells, platelets, or white blood cells other than lymphocytes.

The myeloid and lymphoid stem cells produce colonies of "committed progenitor" cells. Unlike stem cells, committed progenitors are only capable of developing into one specific type of mature cell. Cells passing through the final stages of maturation are called precursor cells.

In healthy human beings, the number of each type of stem cell and their offspring is contained within very narrow limits. Certain proteins, such as interleukins and colony-stimulating factors, play a key role in determining whether a stem cell will replicate itself, produce offspring that evolve into mature blood cells, do both or do neither at any given time. These proteins also regulate the maturation of precursor cells. If this regulatory mechanism breaks down, too many or too few stem cells will be present in the bone marrow and/or certain progenitor or precursor cells will proliferate and fail to properly mature.

In patients with leukemia, for example, one or more types of blood cells (usually white blood cells) fail to properly mature. They stall at one stage of development and self-replicate uncontrollably.

Bone marrow transplants enable physicians to destroy diseased bone marrow with high-dose chemotherapy and/or radiation, and replace it with healthy marrow that will produce normal blood cells. It also enables patients with other malignancies such as breast and ovarian cancer to receive higher than normal doses of chemotherapy to treat their disease. Although the higher doses of chemotherapy destroy bone marrow as well as the tumor, healthy bone marrow can be reinfused after treatment, enabling normal production of blood cells to resume.

CHAPTER 3

Autologous Bone Marrow Transplants

When most people think about bone marrow transplants they envision two parties: the patient who is suffering from a bone marrow disorder such as leukemia, and a bone marrow donor whose healthy bone marrow is used to replace the patient's diseased marrow during transplant. This two-party transplant is called an allogeneic BMT, or syngeneic BMT if the donor is an identical twin.

However another type of BMT, called an autologous (pronounced au-tol´-o-gous) BMT is actually much more common. In an autologous BMT the patient is both the donor and the recipient of the bone marrow. Some 5,000 autologous BMTs are performed each year, outpacing allogeneic and syngeneic BMTs two to one.

Some complications associated with allogeneic BMTs such as graft-versus-host disease are avoided with autologous BMTs. The risk of infection is also somewhat less in autologous BMTs because the large doses of immunosuppressive medications given to patients in allogeneic BMTs to prevent GVHD are not needed.

WHO IS A CANDIDATE FOR AN AUTOLOGOUS BMT

Autologous BMTs (ABMTs) have expanded treatment options for thousands of patients diagnosed with life-threatening diseases such as Hodgkin's disease and non-Hodgkin's lymphoma, breast cancer, ovarian cancer, testicular cancer and pediatric solid tumors such as neuroblastoma. The autologous BMT has also given new hope to hundreds of patients suffering from leukemia who were previously denied a BMT because a suitable bone marrow donor could not be found.

Not all patients diagnosed with these diseases are candidates for an autologous BMT. The type of disease, the stage to which it has progressed, the responsiveness of the disease to prior treatment, and the patient's age and general physical condition are all factors that will

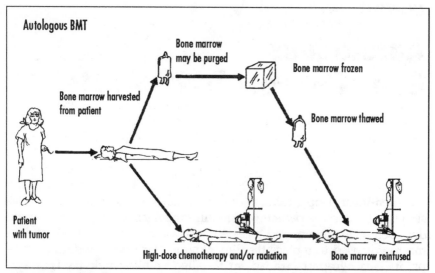

determine whether a patient is considered a suitable candidate for an autologous BMT.

With the exception of leukemia, diseases treated by autologous BMTs are usually not disorders that start in or involve the bone marrow. Rather, they're "malignant" or cancerous tumors located elsewhere in the body that are responsive to treatment with high-dose chemotherapy and/or radiation. The high doses of chemotherapy and/or radiation, however, also destroy the patient's bone marrow. Without bone marrow, the body is unable to manufacture blood cells needed to defend against infection, carry oxygen and prevent bleeding. An autologous BMT enables physicians to "rescue" the patient from the effects of high-dose chemotherapy and/or radiation treatment by replacing the destroyed bone marrow.

For each disease discussed below, long-term survival rates following treatment with an autologous BMT are cited. Keep in mind that these numbers are only ballpark estimates which cover a wide range of circumstances. The projected survival rate of an individual patient will depend on his or her age and general physical condition, the specific characteristics of the disease, the stage to which the disease has progressed, and the responsiveness of the disease to prior treatment. The patient's own physician can provide the best assessment of a patient's chances for long-term survival following an autologous BMT.

Hodgkin's and Non-Hodgkin's Lymphomas

Autologous BMTs are most frequently used to treat patients diagnosed with Hodgkin's disease and non-Hodgkin's lymphoma. In Hodgkin's disease, an abnormal cell called the Reed-Sternberg cell may be present in one or more lymph nodes. Without treatment, this defective cell infiltrates neighboring organs and tissues, disrupting normal functions.

Similarly, in non-Hodgkin's lymphomas, defective lymphocytes (a type of white blood cell) are produced in the lymph nodes, bone marrow, spleen and/or gastrointestinal tract. Left unchecked, they invade other tissues and organs, interfering with their normal functions.

Patients with Hodgkin's disease and non-Hodgkin's lymphoma can often be cured by radiation and/or chemotherapy. However, if patients have not achieved a remission with radiation/chemotherapy, have relapsed after chemotherapy, or have experienced progression of the disease while undergoing chemotherapy, an autologous BMT may be the best option to save their life. Patients with non-Hodgkin's lymphoma whose tumors are not responsive to chemotherapy (ie. the size of the tumor has not shrunk after chemotherapy) are less likely to achieve a long-term cure with an autologous BMT than those whose tumors are responsive to chemotherapy. This is not true for patients with Hodgkin's disease.

Patients with advanced Hodgkin's or non-Hodgkin's lymphoma who undergo an autologous BMT have a 25 to 50 percent chance of long term survival. Without a BMT, their chances for long term survival are 5 to 10 percent.

Leukemia

Treatment of leukemia with an autologous BMT is becoming more common. Patients with acute lymphocytic leukemia (ALL) or acute myelogenous leukemia (AML) (also called acute non-lymphocytic leukemia or ANLL) may be candidates for an autologous BMT if their disease is in complete remission. Since a complete remission is rarely achieved in patients with chronic myelogenous leukemia (CML), an autologous BMT is usually not a treatment option for these patients (although some very interesting studies are now underway using ABMTs to treat this disease).

Leukemia is a disease of the bone marrow, the organ that produces the body's blood cells. In patients with leukemia, a large number of abnormal white blood cells are produced in the bone marrow and interfere with the production of normal blood cells. Without normal blood cells, the body's ability to fight infection, carry oxygen to tissues, and prevent bleeding is impaired. Patients with acute leukemia will die within a matter of weeks or months without treatment.

Patients with acute myelogenous leukemia (AML or ANLL) who've achieved a first complete remission with standard chemotherapy may be able to increase their chances for long-term survival significantly with a BMT. Without a BMT, their expected long-term survival rate is 20 to 30 percent.

Researchers are currently studying whether autologous BMTs are more effective than standard chemotherapy in treating patients with AML in first remission. Preliminary results suggest that survival rates do improve with an autologous BMT, but further study is underway to determine whether these improved survival rates are the result of the autologous BMT or other factors such as the type of patients chosen to participate in the study or the sub-type of AML affecting the patient.

BMTs are also performed on patients with acute lymphocytic leukemia. ALL typically strikes children. Because the cure rate with standard chemotherapy is quite high, only a few studies have been conducted to date on the use of BMTs in the treatment of ALL. While the studies have found that both autologous and allogeneic BMTs are an effective treatment option for ALL patients, some experts believe that too little data are currently available to reliably project long-term survival rates.

People are often surprised that an autologous BMT is a treatment option for patients with leukemia. Since it's known that malignant cells may remain in the bone marrow of patients with leukemia even after a complete remission has been achieved, they question why it makes sense to harvest imperfect marrow and re-infuse it back into the patient via an autologous BMT.

Researchers are not sure of the answer, but some theorize that the number of malignant cells re-introduced into the patient is so small that the body's normal defenses can destroy them before they proliferate. Many centers purge the harvested bone marrow to reduce the number of cancerous cells that remain in the sample. For more information on purging see page 30.

Breast Cancer

Breast cancer is the third most common cancer in women, resulting in thousands of deaths annually. In 1990, 150,000 new cases were diagnosed and 44,000 deaths from breast cancer were reported.

The initial treatment for breast cancer is surgery with or without radiation. In cases where the risk of relapse is high, chemotherapy has sometimes been administered after surgery. However, once breast cancer has spread or become metastatic (Stage IV) it is no longer curable with conventional treatment.

Over the past five years, researchers have been studying the possibility of treating advanced stage breast cancer with a combination of high-dose chemotherapy and an autologous BMT. Since an autologous BMT enables a physician to replace the patient's bone marrow after the chemotherapy treatment, higher doses of chemotherapy can be used than previously possible.

The results of early clinical studies in which high-dose chemotherapy and an autologous BMT were administered to Stage IV breast cancer patients who had previously undergone intensive chemotherapy treatment were encouraging. A remission was achieved in 27 percent of the patients. That remission, however, was of short duration.

Subsequent studies conducted with patients who had just become Stage IV, had not previously undergone intensive chemotherapy treatment or were in their first relapse after remission, found that administering a cycle of chemotherapy before the high-dose chemotherapy and an autologous BMT produced remissions in 50 percent or more of the cases, with some remissions lasting three years or more.

Studies are now underway to determine whether chemotherapy followed by high-dose chemotherapy and an autologous BMT will improve the survival rates of some Stage II breast cancer patients (in whom the disease has spread to lymph nodes under the arm) and some Stage III patients who are in a first remission and have not yet relapsed, but are in a high risk category for relapse (i.e. the disease has spread to 10 or more lymph nodes). Early results from the studies are encouraging.

Childhood Neuroblastoma

Childhood neuroblastoma is a cancer affecting the nerves that run from the neck down the inside of the back to the pelvis. It occurs almost exclusively in very young children. Radiation and surgery are used to treat the disease in early stages when it's localized, but chemotherapy has so far not cured more than a very small percentage of patients when the disease is widespread at diagnosis.

Researchers have attempted to increase the cure rate with high-dose chemotherapy and an autologous BMT. Studies have found that for patients in first remission whose tumor has become resistant to standard chemotherapy, 40-50 percent can achieve a remission lasting two years or more with high-dose chemotherapy and/or total body irradiation and an autologous BMT. Survival rates are not as favorable for patients undergoing an autologous BMT after a relapse. Long-term survival rates for patients treated with an autologous BMT are similar to results achieved with an allogeneic BMT.

Other Diseases

Ovarian cancer, brain tumors, Ewing's Sarcoma, testicular cancer, and other solid tumor cancers may also be treated with autologous BMTs. Ask your doctor for information about the effectiveness of treating these diseases with an autologous BMT.

PURGING BONE MARROW

Purging is a technique used at some transplant centers to reduce the number of cancerous cells that may be in bone marrow harvested from certain patients undergoing an autologous BMT. The theory behind purging is simple: by reducing the number of cancerous cells in the harvested bone marrow, the likelihood of relapse after an autologous BMT will be reduced.

Two different purging techniques are used. The first involves "monoclonal antibodies"—special proteins that distinguish malignant cells from normal cells and attach to the surface of the malignant cell. These "marked" malignant cells are then broken apart with additional proteins called "complement" or "immunotoxins." Alternatively, small magnetic beads or "microspheres" are coated with the monoclonal antibodies and mixed with the bone marrow. The marrow is then passed over electromagnets which remove the microspheres and malignant cells to which they've become attached.

A second technique is chemical or pharmacological purging. The bone marrow is incubated with chemicals more toxic to cancerous cells than normal cells. The marrow is then transplanted into the patient.

Most U.S. transplant centers now purge bone marrow harvested from patients with leukemia before an autologous transplant. Tests on animals have shown purging to be effective in removing leukemic cells that linger in the marrow. Recent European studies suggest a link between purging and improved long-term survival rates in this patient population.

Purging bone marrow harvested from patients with non-Hodgkin's lymphomas is more controversial. No studies to date have conclusively demonstrated that purging bone marrow improves the long-term survival for this group of patients.

Purging is generally not done on bone marrow harvested from patients with Hodgkin's disease. It's commonly done, however, on the bone marrow of patients with neuroblastoma.

Purging has its drawbacks. Pharmacological purging can damage normal as well as malignant cells, causing delayed engraftment of platelets and granulocytes and extending the period in the hospital during which patients are susceptible to infection and bleeding. Problems associated with pharmacological purging are diminishing as researchers learn the optimal level of chemicals to use in the purging procedure.

POST-RECOVERY

The prognosis for long-term survival varies according to the disease being treated, the stage of the disease at which an autologous BMT was performed, the patient's age, prior treatment history, and any complications that may have developed during transplant. There is no guarantee that an autologous BMT (or any BMT for that matter) will cure the disease.

Nonetheless, the alternative is usually near-certain death. Each added day of life, therefore, is special. Most patients agree that the potential rewards of an autologous BMT are well worth the effort.

I was first diagnosed with breast cancer in February 1989. I've since endured 18 months of non-stop treatment including six surgeries, eight weeks of radiation, and finally in March 1990, an autologous BMT. It's hard to believe all I have gone through to fight breast cancer.

I decided to have an autologous BMT as soon as I learned my breast cancer was Stage IV. I felt that chemotherapy would not be adequate to combat the spread of my disease.

A close friend had a BMT for metastatic breast cancer, as did the daughter-in-law of my mother's friend. Both died after their transplants, but their disease was in a more advanced stage than mine when their BMTs were performed. I realized I was doing a very gutsy thing, with two negative role models, and no positive ones for encouragement. But I felt that the fact that my disease was less advanced would make a difference, so I decided to have an autologous BMT right away. What a horrible decision to face, but what a horrible disease!

When I raised the idea of a BMT with my oncology team they were very supportive and stood behind me as I took this shot at a possible cure. I strongly feel that patients should be told about the BMT option when their breast cancer advances to Stage III. Perhaps their chance for a successful transplant would improve if the BMT is done earlier rather than later.

Taking local radiation for the regional spread of my cancer during Phase III did not do the job for me.

Five months after the transplant I was delighted to hear that the doctors could find no evidence of the disease in my body. Even though I felt like I had "just landed" in the first few months after transplant, I was glad I'd decided to have the BMT.

It takes a while to recover emotionally, physically, and psychologically after fighting breast cancer so hard and so long. I feel much better now, despite the heavy assault on my body during treatment.

I used to teach 45 piano students each week. During my battle with breast cancer, however, I could only teach a few students in an intermittent way. Though I've gradually come back to my regular life style, it's very moderate compared to before. It's difficult to strike the balance between the amount of activity that is "enough" to satisfy my mental health, and "too much" given my physical condition.

This ordeal has certainly been the toughest challenge of my life, but I thank God and am proud of myself for coming through it as well as I have. In March I'll have my one year post-transplant check-up. If it's good I'll be dancing on top of the Sears Tower with joy. If it's bad I'll be sad, but I'll know that I chose the most aggressive treatment available to fight my metastatic breast cancer.

"Hats off" to the medical profession and all the doctors who helped save my life; and to all the brave people who cherish life and love enough to attempt a BMT to cure their disease.

Georgia Comfort, age 40, Illinois

Editor's note: Georgia passed her one year post-transplant check-up with flying colors!

CHAPTER 4

Allogeneic Bone Marrow Transplants

Between 1981 and 1990, the number of allogeneic BMTs performed annually worldwide grew six-fold, from 875 in 1981 to 5,529 in 1990. That number is expected to increase by at least 2,000 in 1992.

Allogeneic BMTs are used most frequently to treat patients with leukemia, aplastic anemia and immune deficiency diseases. They differ from autologous BMTs in that the bone marrow donor and patient are two different people.

Despite the increasing number of BMTs performed annually, 60 to 70 percent of patients who need an allogeneic BMT each year go without one because a suitable bone marrow donor can't be found. Although a sibling is usually the preferred bone marrow donor, not every patient has a brother or sister with "matching" bone marrow. Thus, transplants using unrelated donors and "mis-matched" donors are often tried.

In the United States, the National Marrow Donor Program (NMDP) is leading the effort to expand the international registry of volunteer bone marrow donors so that more patients in need of a BMT can access this treatment. As of June 1992, more than 600,000 volunteer donors were part of the NMDP registry and as many as 50 bone marrow transplants with unrelated donors were being facilitated each month. A smaller registry called the American Bone Marrow Donor Registry also maintains several thousand

DISEASES FREQUENTLY TREATED WITH ALLOGENEIC BMTS

Aplastic Anemia

Hodgkin's Disease

Leukemia

Myelodysplasia

Non-Hodgkin's Lymphoma

Multiple Myeloma

Osteopetrosis

Severe Combined Immune Deficiency Syndrome (SCIDs)

Thalassemia

Wiskott-Aldrich Syndrome

donor records that can be searched by patients needing a bone marrow donor.

The difficulty in finding a suitable donor lies in the fact that the donor's and patient's "tissue type" must closely match in order for the transplant to be successful. Genetic markers on the surface of white blood cells called HLA-antigens define a person's tissue type. Since these genetic markers are inherited, siblings are much more likely to have similar HLA-antigens than unrelated persons.

There's a 30-35 percent chance that a patient's sibling will be a suitable donor. If a donor must be located in the general population, the chances of finding a match range from one in 1,000 to one in several million, depending on the frequency of the patient's tissue type in the general population.

THE HLA SYSTEM

Everyone has distinguishing physical characteristics inherited from their parents. Some, such as eye and hair color, are easily seen by the naked eye. Others, such as fingerprints and blood type, require more sophisticated technology to detect.

White blood cells carry a distinguishing "fingerprint" on their surface called the HLA system—the human leukocyte antigen system. (Leukocyte means white blood cell). These antigens are proteins that play a critical role in protecting the body against invading organisms

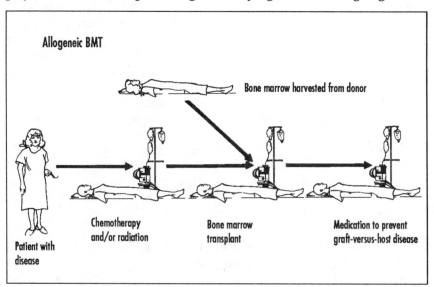

Allogeneic BMT

Bone marrow harvested from donor

Patient with disease

Chemotherapy and/or radiation

Bone marrow transplant

Medication to prevent graft-versus-host disease

such as bacteria, viruses and other foreign matter.

At birth, certain white blood cells called T-cells are programmed by the thymus gland to identify all the antigens that belong in that person's body. When a foreign antigen is encountered, e.g. antigens on the cell surface of invading bacteria or viruses, the T-cells summon the various components of the immune system to attack and destroy the invading organism.

Similarly, when bone marrow is transplanted from a donor into a BMT patient, the patient's T-cells will examine the antigens on cells in the donated marrow, and will launch an immune system attack if they perceive the antigens to be "non-self". If the patient's immune system destroys the donated bone marrow, graft-rejection results and the BMT fails.

Alternatively (and more commonly) the T-cells in the donor's bone marrow overpower the patient's T-cells. They identify the patient's body as "non-self" and orchestrate an immune system attack on the patient's organs. This condition is called graft-versus-host disease (GVHD). (The graft is the donated bone marrow, the host is the patient). GVHD is usually not life-threatening. However, it can be a very uncomfortable side-effect of an allogeneic BMT, and in severe cases can be life-threatening. (See Chapter 9 for more information about GVHD.)

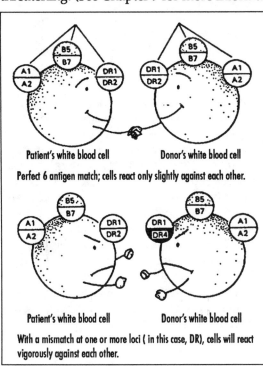

Patient's white blood cell   Donor's white blood cell

Perfect 6 antigen match; cells react only slightly against each other.

Patient's white blood cell   Donor's white blood cell

With a mismatch at one or more loci (in this case, DR), cells will react vigorously against each other.

The HLA fingerprint on white blood cells is composed of a pair of antigens at several sites or "loci" on the white blood cell—one each inherited from the mother and the father. The antigens at three of these sites—the HLA-A, HLA-B, and HLA-DR loci are known to play an important role in determining whether graft-rejection will occur and the severity of GVHD. Pairs of antigens are also known to exist at other sites on white blood cells such as the HLA-C,-E,-DP and DQ-loci. However, their importance in

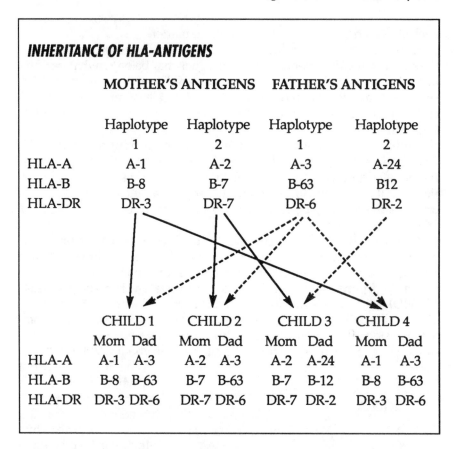

INHERITANCE OF HLA-ANTIGENS

	MOTHER'S ANTIGENS		FATHER'S ANTIGENS	
	Haplotype 1	Haplotype 2	Haplotype 1	Haplotype 2
HLA-A	A-1	A-2	A-3	A-24
HLA-B	B-8	B-7	B-63	B12
HLA-DR	DR-3	DR-7	DR-6	DR-2

	CHILD 1		CHILD 2		CHILD 3		CHILD 4	
	Mom	Dad	Mom	Dad	Mom	Dad	Mom	Dad
HLA-A	A-1	A-3	A-2	A-3	A-2	A-24	A-1	A-3
HLA-B	B-8	B-63	B-7	B-63	B-7	B-12	B-8	B-63
HLA-DR	DR-3	DR-6	DR-7	DR-6	DR-7	DR-2	DR-3	DR-6

bone marrow transplantation is not yet fully understood.

To date, 24 different possible antigens have been identified at the HLA-A site, 52 at the HLA-B site, and 20 at the HLA-DR site. Since each person has two antigens at each site, more than 600 million combinations of HLA antigens are theoretically possible in the general population! Fortunately, the antigens at the HLA-A,-B and -DR loci are usually inherited as a set called a "haplotype" from one or both parents, and certain types tend to occur together, thus reducing the number of possible HLA combinations known to occur in the general population.

In the figure above, for example, one of the mother's haplotypes consists of the antigens A-1, B-8, and DR-3; the other consists of the antigens A-2, B-7 and DR-7. Children #1 and #4 have inherited the mother's first haplotype, while children #2 and #3 have inherited the second. Children #1, #2 and #4 have inherited the father's first haplotype, while child #3 inherited the father's second haplotype.

HLA-Matching

To minimize the risk of graft rejection and graft-versus-host disease, a donor whose HLA type matches that of the patient is best. The optimal donor is often an identical twin. Not only will the twin have inherited from the father and mother the same antigens at the major loci (HLA-A, -B, and -DR) as the patient, but the antigens at tissue antigen sites other than HLA sites that are more difficult to detect or whose role in transplantation is unclear will also match. The risk of either graft-rejection or severe GVHD in BMTs using marrow from an identical twin is eliminated.

In other cases, the best bone marrow donor will be a sibling who is not an identical twin, but whose HLA-A, -B, and -DR antigens match those of the patient. In the figure on page 36, for example, Child #1 and Child #4 are a "perfect" HLA match, having each inherited one identical haplotype from their father and one identical haplotype from their mother. There may, however, be some mis-match at other less significant or well understood non-HLA loci which can cause mild to severe graft-versus-host disease post transplant. The risk of developing severe GVHD in a transplant using a matched sibling donor is approximately 20 percent, and the risk of graft rejection is usually less than 1 percent.

Child #2 and Child #3, on the other hand, each inherited an identical haplotype from their mother, but different haplotypes from their father. Were Child #2 or Child #3 to need a bone marrow transplant, either an unrelated bone marrow donor with matching antigens at the HLA-A, -B, and -DR loci would have to be found, or a transplant using "mismatched" bone marrow from their sibling would have to be considered.

HLA-Typing Tests

At least two tests are used to determine whether a patient's and donor's HLA-types match. The first is a blood test that can detect antigens at the HLA-A, -B and -DR loci. Secondary tests, such as the mixed lymphocyte culture (MLC) test, are used to assess whether or not the patient's and donor's bone marrow interact adversely.

Newer tests such as DNA typing will make HLA-typing more precise in the future. DNA testing has already revealed that antigens once thought to be identical may in fact have as many as 10 different variations or "microvariants". The significance of all these variations is not yet known, but they may explain the increased frequency and intensity of GVHD and occurrence of graft rejection in BMTs using mis-matched or unrelated donors.

MATCHED RELATED DONORS

Between 1988 and 1990, approximately 12,000 allogeneic BMTS with matched related donors were performed worldwide, according to data compiled by the International Bone Marrow Transplant Registry. Forty-seven percent involved patients with acute leukemias, 27 percent were performed on patients with chronic leukemias, 10 percent on patients with lymphomas and other cancers, 9 percent on patients with aplastic anemia, and the remainder on patients with thalassemia, immune deficiency disorders and genetic or metabolic storage diseases.

Acute Myelogenous Leukemia (AML)

Acute myelogenous leukemia (also called acute non-lymphocytic leukemia or ANLL) is a class of leukemias that includes acute myeloblastic leukemia (M1), acute myelocytic leukemia (M2, also called acute granulocytic leukemia), acute promyelocytic leukemia (M3), acute myelomonocytic leukemia (M4), acute monocytic leukemia (M5), acute erythroleukemia (M6), and acute megakaryocytic leukemia (M7). Most patients with AML who undergo an allogeneic BMT do so while in first remission.

When first diagnosed, patients with AML are given a cycle of chemotherapy called "induction chemotherapy" to achieve a remission (i.e., no leukemic cells can be seen when bone marrow is examined under a microscope). However, undetected leukemic cells usually persist following induction chemotherapy, and 80 percent of patients eventually relapse without further treatment.

To improve the cure rate, induction chemotherapy is usually followed by another cycle of chemotherapy called consolidation chemotherapy, or by an allogeneic BMT. The cure rate with consolidation chemotherapy is 30 percent for adults, and 40 to 50 percent for children. The cure rate for those undergoing an allogeneic BMT in first remission is 50 percent for adults (some single institutions have reported cure rates as high as 65 percent), and 60 to 80 percent for children.

If a patient fails to achieve remission following induction chemotherapy, or if the patient relapses (the leukemia comes back) following consolidation chemotherapy, an allogeneic BMT may still be possible. Under these circumstances, the chances for long-term survival are 10 to 30 percent. Without a BMT, the chances are 0 to 5 percent.

Some patients with AML who lack an HLA-matched donor, and thus are unable to have an allogeneic BMT, undergo an autologous BMT with purged marrow. (See Chapter 3 for more on autologous BMTs and marrow purging.)

Acute Lymphocytic Leukemia (ALL)

Acute lymphocytic leukemia (ALL) is the most common form of leukemia in children and is highly curable with conventional chemotherapy. Bone marrow transplantation is usually reserved for those who do not achieve a remission, or for those who relapse.

Approximately 30 to 40 percent of ALL patients who undergo an allogeneic BMT while in second remission are cured of their disease. Without a BMT, the chances for long-term survival among those who relapse or do not achieve a first remission are 0 to 5 percent.

Studies have been conducted to determine whether undergoing an allogeneic BMT while in first remission improves the cure rate for certain "high risk" ALL patients (i.e., patients at high risk of relapse following standard chemotherapy because of age, high white blood cell count, etc.). Preliminary results suggest that cure rates as high as 50 to 70 percent may be achieved for this subset of patients, versus a 30 percent cure rate with standard chemotherapy. Further studies are underway to verify these promising results.

Chronic Myelogenous Leukemia (CML)

Chronic myelogenous leukemia (also called chronic granulocytic leukemia) is a form of leukemia that progresses more slowly than AML or ALL. It is often controllable for years with hydroxyurea or interferon. Eventually, however, CML reaches an acute stage in which the disease progresses rapidly, and death occurs without intensive therapy.

For patients who undergo an allogeneic BMT early in the course of their disease (during the first year of diagnosis appears to be optimal), the cure rate is 50 to 80 percent. Those who wait until the leukemia progresses to the acute stage have a cure rate of 10 to 30 percent.

Hodgkin's and Non-Hodgkin's Lymphomas

Typically, patients with Hodgkin's disease and non-Hodgkin's lymphomas who cannot be cured with conventional chemotherapy undergo an autologous BMT rather than an allogeneic BMT (see Chapter 3). However, if the disease has spread/to the bone marrow, an allogeneic BMT may be the best or only chance for a cure. For this subset of patients, the long-term survival rate following an allogeneic BMT is 20 percent, as compared to 0 to 5 percent with standard chemotherapy.

Aplastic Anemia

In patients with aplastic anemia, the bone marrow malfunctions, resulting in low white blood cell, red blood cell and platelet counts. Therefore, patients with aplastic anemia are very susceptible to infection and bleeding.

An allogeneic BMT is the preferred treatment for younger patients with an HLA-matched donor. Fifty to 70 percent of patients achieve normal blood counts following an allogeneic BMT.

For older patients and those who lack a suitable bone marrow donor, antithymocyte globulin (ATG), used alone or in combination with steroids and cyclosporine, can successfully treat the disease in 50 percent of cases. ATG is used to destroy T-cells which may cause aplastic anemia in certain patients. If this treatment fails, an allogeneic BMT remains an option.

MIS-MATCHED BMTS

Since the chances of finding a donor among one's siblings are only 30 to 35 percent (given the current family size of 2.7 children) trials have been underway to determine whether partially matched or "mis-matched" related donors can be used effectively in BMTs. Results to date indicate that a sibling mis-matched for one antigen at either the HLA-A,-B or -DR site (a 5 out of 6 antigen match) can often be a suitable bone marrow donor.

In transplants using single antigen mis-matched related donors, the risk of developing severe graft-versus-host disease is approximately 30 percent (as compared to 20 percent in HLA-matched related transplants). The risk of graft-rejection is approximately 10 percent. Despite the higher risk of severe GVHD in one-antigen mis-matched related transplants, the long-term survival rate is approximately the same as that seen in BMTs using HLA-matched related donors.

When more than one antigen in the donated bone marrow is mis-matched, the risk of developing severe graft-versus-host disease is 50 to 70 percent, and long-term survival rates decrease markedly for most types of patients.

Use of mis-matched related donors has been successful in BMTs for patients with immune deficiency diseases such as SCIDs (severe combined immune deficiency syndrome). A three-antigen mis-matched parent (or 3 out of 6 antigen match) can often serve as a donor for these patients. Since immune deficient patients have no functioning immune system, they are usually incapable of launching an immune system attack on the donated bone marrow and thus the incidence of graft-rejection is very low. New techniques to remove the T-cells from the donor's marrow (the cells believed responsible for causing graft-versus-disease) have reduced the incidence and severity of GVHD in this patient population.

Patients with severe aplastic anemia have responded least favorably to BMTs using mis-matched donors. Graft-rejection rates as high as 40-50 percent have been reported, but these numbers are less if the BMT preparative regimen includes total body irradiation. The high graft rejection rate may be partly due to the large number of transfusions many aplastic anemia patients receive prior to a BMT, which make the patient more sensitive to antigens on cells in the donor's bone marrow.

In patients with leukemia, transplants using single-antigen mis-matched related donors have produced long-term survival results similar to those obtained when marrow from an HLA-matched sibling is used, despite a higher incidence of GVHD and graft rejection. If more than one antigen is mis-matched however, the incidence of severe graft-versus-host disease increases significantly, and long-term survival rates fall. Although T-cell depletion techniques reduce the incidence of graft-versus-host disease, they also increase the rate of graft rejection in this patient population because T-cells are needed for engraftment. Thus, the overall survival rates have remained unchanged. Patients in an advanced stage of leukemia who must receive higher dosages of chemotherapy and/or radiation than others prior to their transplant have the greatest risk of developing life-threatening GVHD when mis-matched related bone marrow is used.

While BMTs using bone marrow from a single-antigen mis-matched related donor are often successful, this does not significantly expand the pool of potential donors for most patients. The chance of finding a family member mis-matched for one HLA-antigen is only 3 to 5 percent. Thus, efforts are underway to expand the international registry of unrelated bone marrow donors.

UNRELATED DONOR TRANSPLANTS

Bone marrow donor registries now exist in more than 30 countries, with over 750,000 potential bone marrow donors on file. Currently, 70 hospitals in the United States perform allogeneic BMTs with unrelated bone marrow donors.

The likelihood of finding a matched unrelated donor among the general population depends on a number of factors. The first is the patient's haplotypes—the two sets of HLA antigens inherited from his or her parents. If the haplotypes are fairly common, the chance of finding a matched donor in the current NMDP registry of 600,000 donors is quite good. Patients with very rare haplotypes, on the other hand, may have less than a 10 percent chance of finding a matched donor.

The second factor is the patient's ethnic group. Some HLA-antigens are "pan-ethnic," i.e. they are found among members of nearly every ethnic group. Other HLA-antigens are found more frequently in members of a specific ethnic group. If a patient's antigens are more commonly found in one ethnic group than others, his or her ability to find a matched donor will be limited by the number of members of that ethnic group in the donor registry. For this reason, efforts are underway to expand the ethnic diversity of donors in the NMDP registry.

The third factor is the patient's diagnosis and stage of disease. Searching for an unrelated donor can take 3-10 months, sometimes years. Patients with a rapidly progressing disease are at a disadvantage when searching for an unrelated donor, because of the long turn-around time currently required to locate a matching donor. This is sometimes the reason that a mis-matched related donor is used.

Since the first BMT with an unrelated donor was attempted in 1973, several studies have shown that a BMT using an unrelated donor is an effective treatment for certain patients diagnosed with leukemia, aplastic anemia, and immune deficiency syndromes. More work needs to be done, however, to enable more precise matching of donors with patients, and to minimize the incidence and severity of graft-versus-host disease.

Research is underway at some BMT centers to determine the feasibility of using mis-matched unrelated donors in BMTs. Preliminary studies indicate that a BMT using a single antigen mis-matched (or a 5 out of 6 antigen match) unrelated donor can be successful, but the risk of severe GVHD is very high. The results tend to be better when the patient is a child, rather than an adult. If no donor is available, some patients may be candidates for an autologous BMT (See Chapter 3).

SEARCHING FOR AN UNRELATED DONOR

The National Marrow Donor Program (NMDP) maintains the largest database of donors in the United States. As of June 1992, more than 600,000 volunteer donor records could be accessed through the NMDP registry.

The NMDP conducts a donor search for individual patients only at the request of an authorized NMDP transplant center. Authorized centers are those that have performed 10 or more allogeneic transplants per year in the last two years and 30 in the last five years. Phone the NMDP at 800-654-1247 for a current list of NMDP authorized transplant centers and their criteria for accepting patients.

A smaller registry of bone marrow donors, the American Registry, reported 40,000 donors on file as of June 1992, with access to several hundred thousand international records as well. Most of the international records can also be accessed through the NMDP.

Any physician or transplant center can initiate a donor search of the American Registry. If the patient is over 50 years of age, the donor search must be requested by a transplant center willing to perform the transplant. For information on searching the American Registry's donor database call 800-726-2824.

Charges for searching the NMDP and American Registry databases vary, depending on the number of potential donors identified and follow-up tests that must be performed. Fees for the donor search, donor blood tests, physical exam of the donor, and bone marrow harvest can be as much as $20,000. Not all insurance plans cover these donor-related costs.

BEING A DONOR

If a person is called upon to serve as a bone marrow donor, the medical procedure he or she must undergo is called a bone marrow harvest. It is a surgical procedure that typically requires one overnight stay in the hospital. The procedure is generally performed under general anesthesia so the donor feels no discomfort while the bone marrow is being harvested. Afterwards, the donor may feel some soreness in the hip area where the bone marrow was withdrawn. This soreness can usually be relieved by taking oral medications like Tylenol. For a more detailed explanation of a bone marrow harvest, see page 13.

If you have volunteered to be a bone marrow donor through the National Marrow Donor Program or the American Registry, the costs associated with donating bone marrow are typically covered by the patient's family. Bone marrow donors can expect to spend approximately 40 hours (cumulatively, not consecutively) on the various blood tests, physical exams, counseling sessions and the bone marrow harvest itself. If you are a related donor, you will probably also be asked to serve as the patient's platelet donor during the first few weeks following the BMT.

For most donors, the opportunity to give a person, especially a loved one, a second chance at life is very exciting. Keep in mind, however, that not all BMTs are successful. News of an unsuccessful transplant can be very hard on a donor who's made a substantial physical and emotional investment in saving another person's life. Donors can only be guaranteed that they'll give the patient "a future." Whether that future is two months, two years or a lifetime cannot be predicted with certainty.

F orty-year-old Laura Wise of Illinois is a typical mother. At the first sign of illness, she hustles her three children and husband off to the doctor. But in the Spring of 1990, when flu-like symptoms started bothering her, she put off a call to the doctor for months.

When she went for a check-up she was stunned by the news. She had chronic myelogenous leukemia. With conventional treatment, her doctor predicted she had 3-5 years to live.

"It felt like a death sentence" Laura recalls "but fortunately my doctor gave me exactly what I needed right from the start: hope. He explained that a bone marrow transplant might possibly cure me and suggested we begin testing my two sisters and brother immediately to see if one of them could be a donor. Deciding to have the transplant was hard, but once I made the decision I never looked back."

Waiting for the HLA test results on her sisters and brother was even harder. "There was such a sense of urgency to proceed with the transplant, yet it seemed like an eternity before the test results were finally in. At first I didn't really understand what they meant. I'd look at them and think 'This is pretty good. They're only a couple of antigens off!' "

As is often the case, none of Laura's siblings was a perfect HLA-match. Her sister Mary was the closest—a one-antigen mis-match—and her doctors decided she would be an acceptable donor.

In August, Laura, her husband Bob and Mary travelled to Seattle for the transplant. "It was hard leaving our three children behind, but we wanted their life to be as normal as possible during the BMT. All three (ages 4-9) had a sense of what was happening and we phoned them every day."

Mary's "marvelous marrow" engrafted without problem and her "powerful platelets" sustained Laura until she was able to produce platelets on her own. She did, however, develop chronic GVHD after being discharged from the hospital.

"I've had a skin rash, mouth sores, dry itching eyes and elevated liver functions, and have been taking cyclosporine to control it. At my one year check-up last August, I started tapering off the drugs. Six weeks later, the GVHD flared up and I had to go back on cyclosporine. That was disappointing."

Since then, Laura's GVHD has subsided. "This July I'll have another check-up. Hopefully I can taper off the drugs and the GVHD will finally fizzle out."

"For me, the transplant was totally worth it. For the most part, I'm back to a normal routine."

Her suggestion for new BMT patients: "Always look on the hopeful side of things. That, and the wonderful support given to me by my husband and family made all the difference in the world in getting me through the experience."

CHAPTER 5

Peripheral Stem Cell Transplants

In 1991, an estimated 1,000 U.S. patients underwent a peripheral stem cell harvest (PSCH) and transplant. PSCHs have been used instead of or in addition to autologous bone marrow harvests when transplanting patients with acute myelogenous leukemia (AML, also called acute non-lymphocytic leukemia or ANLL), acute lymphocytic leukemia (ALL), Hodgkin's disease, non-Hodgkin's lymphoma, brain tumors, breast cancer, ovarian cancer, multiple myeloma, small cell lung cancer, testicular cancer and neuroblastoma.

More than 58 BMT centers in the U.S. now perform peripheral stem cell harvests and transplants and that number is growing. Peripheral stem cell transplants differ from autologous BMTs only in the method of collecting "stem cells," the cells that are reinfused into the patient during the transplant.

STEM CELLS

Mature blood cells evolve from "mother" cells called stem cells. The most primitive of these is the pluripotent stem cell that is believed to be the origin of all blood cells.

Pluripotent stem cells differ from other blood cells in that they are capable both of unlimited self-renewal and differentiation. Self-renewal means the cell is able to reproduce another cell identical to itself, thus maintaining a steady number of these types of cells in the body. Differentiation means the cell is capable of generating one or more subsets of more mature cells that eventually evolve into either erythrocytes, neutrophils, eosinophils, basophils, lymphocytes, monocytes or platelets.

When physicians harvest bone marrow for use in a transplant, it is the stem cells they are seeking. Stem cells resemble medium sized white blood cells. It has been estimated that less than one in 100,000 cells in the bone marrow are stem cells.

When stem cells are infused into a patient's bloodstream, they will migrate to the interior of certain bones, set up housekeeping or "colonize" and begin producing immature cells called "committed progenitors." These committed progenitors produce colonies of cells that eventually mature into red blood cells, white blood cells, or platelets.

Although the largest concentration of stem cells in the body is found in the bone marrow, stem cells also can be found in the bloodstream or "peripheral blood." The concentration of stem cells in the bloodstream is normally 1/100 of that in bone marrow. Extracting stem cells from the peripheral blood is called a "peripheral stem cell harvest" or PSCH.

PERIPHERAL STEM CELL HARVEST

The process used to extract stem cells from the bloodstream is similar to the process used to collect platelets from platelet donors. Patients are connected to a cell separation machine or "apheresis" device. A needle is inserted in each arm and blood is withdrawn from one arm and circulated through the machine to extract the stem cells. The remaining cells are returned to the patient through a needle in the opposite arm. Alternatively, the blood may be withdrawn and returned to the patient through a catheter.

DISEASES TREATED WITH PSC TRANSPLANTS

Acute Leukemias

Brain Tumors

Breast Cancer

Hodgkin's Disease

Multiple Myeloma

Neuroblastoma

Non-Hodgkin's Lymphomas

Ovarian Cancer

Sarcoma

Testicular Cancer

The PSCH is painless. Patients occasionally experience lightheadedness, coldness, numbness around the lips, or cramping in the hands during the harvest.

Typically, several two-to-six-hour sessions are required to collect sufficient stem cells from the bloodstream for transplantation. If drugs called "growth factors" or "colony-stimulating factors" (e.g., granulocyte-colony stimulating factor, G-CSF, or granulocyte-macrophage colony stimulating factor, GM-CSF) are given before and during the period of time when peripheral stem cells are being harvested, the number and duration of the sessions may be less. The procedure is usually performed on an outpatient basis over a one- to two-week period. After each session, the stem

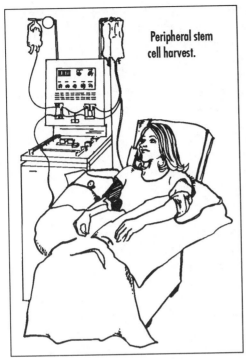

Peripheral stem cell harvest.

cells are frozen using a process called cryopreservation.

REASONS FOR PSCHS

Physicians may recommend a PSCH for a variety of reasons. Sometimes PSCHs are used to augment the stem cells collected from a bone marrow harvest. In other cases, a patient's bone marrow may be contaminated by cancerous cells and a PSCH may be used in lieu of a bone marrow harvest in the hope that the peripheral blood stem cells have not been similarly contaminated. Prior radiation to the pelvic area or chemotherapy can also reduce the number of stem cells available via a bone marrow harvest, making a PSCH necessary.

PROS AND CONS OF PSCHS

A PSCH may provide patients whose bone marrow is unsuitable for harvesting their only opportunity to undergo an autologous transplant. PSCH also allows collection of stem cells without the use of general anesthesia, involves little or no discomfort and can be done on an outpatient basis.

Collection of stem cells through a PSCH, however, requires many days or even weeks while bone marrow harvests can be completed in a single two-hour session in an operating room. The difference in time required to harvest stem cells from the peripheral blood vs. the bone marrow may be critical for patients whose disease is progressing rapidly.

PSCHs also require more laboratory processing time since each sample must be frozen separately. This may increase costs and/or strain laboratory resources at some centers. In a 1992 BMT Newsletter survey of

58 BMT centers performing PSCHs, 38 percent said PSCHs cost more than bone marrow harvests to obtain sufficient stem cells for transplantation. Thirty-one percent said the difference in cost was greater than 20 percent.

Although stem cells derived from the bloodstream can be successfully used in an autologous transplant, they do not appear to be exactly the same as stem cells derived from bone marrow. Whether the stem cells used in a transplant are collected from the bone marrow or peripheral blood, however, does not appear to affect the incidence of full recovery or rate of long term survival. Ultimately, the success of an autologous BMT depends less on the source of stem cells used in the transplant than on the effectiveness of the chemotherapy and/or radiation administered to destroy the diseased cells before the transplant.

F orty-six-year-old Thelda D. of Indiana has lots to be proud of. Less than a year after undergoing a peripheral stem cell harvest and transplant to treat her breast cancer, she's back to work full time, enjoying her first grandchild, Erin, and helping others who face the prospect of a bone marrow transplant.

For Thelda, the road to recovery wasn't easy. At first, Blue Cross/Blue Shield refused to pay for her treatment. "When the women at the school where I work heard about the denial they were very concerned," said Thelda. "They knew the same thing could happen to them." With the help of a letter writing campaign orchestrated by school employees and neighbors, the intervention of Indiana State Representative Kent Adams and former Governor Otis Bowen, and the work of an attorney, Blue Cross/Blue Shield finally relented and agreed to pay.

For eight consecutive days in April 1991, Thelda and her husband Larry drove the five-hour round trip to Chicago and back for the peripheral stem cell harvest. "The nurses were real angels of mercy," said Thelda. "One even fixed us home cooked meals and brought movies to keep us entertained during the harvest."

Meanwhile, friends and neighbors in their townheld a dance and other fundraisers to help with expenses. Larry, a truck driver, had been laid off since Christmas and turned down the chance to return to work in the spring so he could be with Thelda during treatment. In June, 28 days after being admitted to the hospital for the transplant, Thelda arrived home.

"The support I got from family, friends, and the community while I was hospitalized was unreal," said Thelda. "My 70-year-old parents, my son and his friends, and other family members all made the long drive to visit me. The school principal and teachers came to donate platelets. When my daughter, who was five months pregnant visited, I was really inspired to get well. I wanted to see my first grandchild."

Thelda was back to work full time at the end of July. "The first week was hard—I barely had the energy to eat and go to bed when I got home. But it got better with each day that passed."

Before long, Thelda had a chance to repay the kindness she experienced during her treatment. "A 64-year-old man from a nearby community kept following my progress and asking about me," she said. "I finally found out he was going to have a peripheral stem cell transplant for lymphoma in Indianapolis, so I wrote to give him encouragement." They met for the first time a month ago and have been giving each other support ever since. "When you give a little of yourself, you get a lot back in return."

"Deciding to have a transplant is not easy," says Thelda. "At first you feel like you're on a roller coaster. Everything's out of control. Your life's in the hands of strangers and there's a tremendous fear of the unknown. Sometimes my mind was a blank and other times I wondered 'What am I doing?' But then I thought 'What's the alternative? If I'm going to die, I want to go down fighting.' I wasn't ready to give in to the disease. I feel special to be a survivor."

CHAPTER 6

Emotional and Psychological Considerations

A bone marrow transplant (BMT) provides hope for many patients diagnosed with leukemia, aplastic anemia, and other bone marrow disorders and cancers that were once thought incurable. This hope for a cure sustains patients and their families through the difficult period of treatment and recovery. Nonetheless, contemplating a bone marrow transplant, undergoing the procedure and coping with the recovery process is a trying experience for the patient, the patient's family and friends.

COPING WITH THE NEWS

When a patient first faces the prospect of a bone marrow transplant, the news can be devastating. Many will not yet have come to grips with the fact that they're suffering from a life-threatening disease before being asked to decide whether or not to undergo a bone marrow transplant. Sometimes the decision must be made quickly to provide the greatest likelihood of success, adding more stress to an already difficult situation.

The sheer volume of information patients must absorb coupled with their unfamiliarity with the medical jargon used to describe the procedures can be mind-numbing. Some simply stop hearing new information as they struggle to deal with facts already provided and the prospect of their own mortality. Patients may ask the same question repeatedly, failing each time to comprehend the answer.

Little of the information BMT patients receive will sound like good news. What patients want to hear is that the bone marrow transplant will be a quick, painless, risk-free procedure. More importantly, they want assurance that it will cure their disease and provide them with many extra years of life. Unfortunately, no such assurance can be given. The patient can only be promised the "chance" of a future.

Fear that more unsettling news is forthcoming precludes many patients from asking questions. As much as they may want answers, some opt to cope with uncertainty rather than open themselves up to more disturbing news.

GETTING INFORMATION

In an effort to provide a complete and honest description of the BMT experience, doctors sometimes confuse and overwhelm patients. They may assume that patients are familiar with medical jargon like "catheters, IVs, aspirates, biopsies, etc." which is usually not the case. As one patient put it "doctors talk medical, patients talk human".

Don't be embarrassed to ask your doctor to re-explain something or to translate it into words that you can understand. Keep asking questions until you're satisfied with the answer, regardless of how many repetitions it takes.

Ask your doctor to help you put the complications and side effects associated with a BMT into perspective. Don't assume that the likelihood of death or severe liver damage, for example, is as great as the likelihood of temporary hair loss or mouth sores. (It's not!) Ask what the probability is that various complications will occur. It can help ease your worries.

Doctors also sometimes forget to mention that pain relief will be provided during a BMT. Thus, when patients hear about the numerous complications that might occur, they presume they'll be in terrible pain while hospitalized. While pain can occur following a BMT, pain medications can be provided in most cases to alleviate the discomfort.

Family and friends can help patients sort through the deluge of information received from a doctor. A patient who's afraid or embarrassed to ask a physician the same question for the tenth time will appreciate a family member who asks the question on his or her behalf. Giving a patient the name of someone who has experienced a bone marrow transplant and is willing to talk about it can also be helpful. Before meeting your your transplant doctor, it helps to write down any questions you might have and bring them with you.

SETTING GOALS

The time spent in the hospital before, during, and after a bone marrow transplant can seem never-ending. Patients seldom make daily

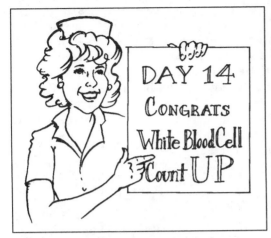

progress by leaps and bounds. Each day will bring a small step forward, maybe a little backsliding, or no change at all. This slow pace of progress can depress patients (and their loved ones) who want desperately to get well and put this chapter of their life behind them.

It helps to take one day at a time rather than worry about what will happen in five days, five weeks or five years. Physicians and health care workers can help by setting manageable goals for patients to achieve each day and by letting them know each and every time progress is made, no matter how small. What the medical staff may take for granted as the normal course of transplant recovery can be big, encouraging news for the patient. When the marrow engrafts, when test results are good, and when blood counts begin to rise, patients should be told and congratulated. Providing the patient with a chart that graphs his or her progress toward the blood count goals can help. Patients constantly feel overwhelmed by "bad" news. Any progress or positive news, no matter how small, can buoy a patient's spirits.

Similarly, encouraging comments from family members on days when a patient looks better can boost the patient's morale. On those inevitable days when backsliding occurs, it's best to discuss your disappointment with someone other than the patient.

LOSS OF CONTROL

A bone marrow transplant is a physically debilitating experience. Patients undergoing a transplant will be in a fragile state of health for several weeks and feel extremely weak and helpless. Walking without assistance, focusing on a book or television set, following the thread of a conversation, or even sitting up in bed may require more energy than the patient has to spare. Patients who are used to being in charge, taking care of themselves, or being the person upon whom others depend will find this physical debilitation very hard to cope with. This loss of control can both frighten and anger a patient.

Two strategies can help to reduce the fear the patient feels during this period. First, patients should be assured that a loved one will be their advocate while they're too weak to fend for themselves. If a patient needs pain relief, has questions, or needs some other form of help, being able to rely on a loved one to track down the appropriate hospital personnel and get the problem solved can be an immense relief. Patients know that physicians and hospital staff have many patients' needs to juggle. Knowing that someone close will be an advocate for the patient, and that patient only, can be very comforting.

Second, patients' fears can be needlessly heightened by a vacuum of information. Isolated in a private room, patients often wonder whether anyone is reviewing their case each day and following up on questions or complaints. Asking physicians, interns, and nurses to touch base frequently with the patient throughout the day, even if there is no new information to report, helps assure patients that they have not been forgotten.

Patients are frequently put in the hands of medical technicians, transport workers or other unfamiliar hospital staff for x-rays and other tests. The fear engendered by their weakened condition is often heightened during these periods. X-ray technicians who handle patients clumsily or leave them stranded on tables for what seems like an eternity, transport workers who manipulate controls on IV lines during transport, etc. can frighten patients who lack the physical strength or medical knowledge to correct a problem if it arises. Similarly, tests that in some way physically restrain a patient, such as those requiring tight-fitting masks on a patient's face, or CAT scans that enclose the patient in a confining space can be frightening. Having a loved one or trusted nurse present during

---

TIPS FOR PATIENTS

- Don't hesitate to ask questions. Sometimes medical personnel assume that you know what's going on when you do not.

- Write things down, especially your questions. During your BMT experience, your memory can be short or unpredictable.

- Ask your doctor for names of former BMT patients with whom you can talk, or a support group you can attend.

- Ask for a tour of the BMT unit and a demonstration of equipment that will be used during your stay before you're admitted to the hospital.

- Take one day at a time.

these procedures, or providing a mild sedative, can calm the patient and alleviate stress.

Patients often react to the loss of control over their body with anger. This anger may be directed at physicians, other medical personnel or even at the patient's loved ones. There are several things care-givers can do to diffuse the patient's anger and frustration.

Most importantly, treat patients with respect. Even in a debilitated state, adult patients want and are entitled to be treated as adults. Their intelligence should be acknowledged, their modesty respected, and their need to assert some control over their own situation understood.

Patients can react angrily to persons who try to "dictate" rather than tactfully encourage them to do things they'd rather not do. Giving the patient a chance to assert some control over these decisions can lessen their feeling of helplessness and anger.

Respecting a patient's modesty and privacy can also stem a source of anger. As sick and helpless as patients may be, there's no reason to require them to bare their bodies and souls to the world.

Patients often need time alone with physicians, psychologists, or social workers to discuss private concerns and feelings. Family members and friends should respect this need. Sitting in on discussions, especially between the patient and psychological or pastoral counselors, may prevent the patient from expressing feelings and concerns with which he or she needs help coping.

ISOLATION

The special precautions taken to protect BMT patients against infection after the transplant while their immune system is suppressed make many patients feel lonely and isolated. Transplant patients crave a normal environment where they're not the center of attention, where they can interact freely with family and friends without special precautions or protective garb, and where they can think about something other than their disease and treatment.

Converting a hospital room into the patient's room can make the patient feel less detached from normal life. Having pictures of family members on hand, displaying cards and well wishes, substituting pictures of the patient's choosing for the "art" that normally adorns hospital room walls helps. Bringing in the patient's own bed clothes, a tape deck with favorite music, books, a VCR, etc. can also make the hospital room seem homier.

When family and friends visit, they should talk about the world outside. Positive, upbeat anecdotes about family members and friends, descriptions of stores or museums visited, plays or movies that have been seen, the latest gossip from work or school—anything that brings the outside world to patients—will make them feel less isolated and cut off from normal life.

PHYSICAL DISCOMFORT

Some side effects of the high-dose chemotherapy and/or radiation patients undergo prior to transplant as well as post-transplant medications and complications can be stressful for patients.

Temporary hair loss can change one's self image, making some patients self-conscious or embarrassed to be seen by family and friends. During the hospital stay, wearing a head scarf, turban, or hat may make a patient feel less conspicuous and can be more comfortable than a wig.

Meals, too, can be a stressful time. Hospital food, even on the best days, can be a pretty miserable bill of fare. Mouth sores, a common side effect of the treatment, can make eating uncomfortable. Some of the drugs administered to patients during treatment may radically alter the taste of foods, making them unpalatable. Patients often appreciate having family members bring in "comfort foods" that are more appealing to the patient (provided they've been approved by the doctor).

The large quantity of medications patients will need to take orally each day can be daunting, and some may have difficulty as they try to force the pills down. The battery of tests administered to monitor the patient's overall physical condition, while not painful, can leave patients feeling like their bodies are under constant assault. Though little can be done to curtail these necessary medications and tests, sympathy from all care-givers can help patients cope with the stress they produce.

In some cases, it is possible to reduce the physical discomfort associated with a test and thus reduce stress. Pre-medication with demerol or morphine prior to a bone marrow aspirate, for example, can calm a patient and make the procedure more comfortable. Patients should not be reticent about asking for pre-medication or other pain relief if they're worried about discomfort. Don't be intimidated if the medical staff seems resistant to your request. There's no reason to endure more pain than necessary.

Families of BMT patients should take an active, aggressive role in advising physicians and hospital staff of a patient's discomfort and needs. Family members know the patient's personality best and will know the extent to which a patient will be stoic about pain and discomfort before asking for help. The hospital staff needs to know if the patient will request relief as soon as pain begins or only after the discomfort is really intense. The speed with which they respond to the patient's call for help is often influenced by this important information.

PSYCHIATRIC HELP

Anxiety and stress are a normal and expected part of the BMT experience. Patients who become very anxious or agitated are not "weaklings" or losing their minds. They're reacting in a very normal way to a very stressful experience.

Most BMT patients benefit from the services of a psychiatrist or psychologist during the BMT process and patients should be encouraged to take advantage of their professional help. If your physician does not volunteer these helpful services to you, ask for them.

Some patients will be shocked or embarrassed at the notion that they may be incapable of coping with the stress of a BMT on their own. This is particularly true of persons who've never before required the help of a psychologist or psychiatrist. Needing and seeking psychological or psychiatric help during a BMT is normal. It does not mean the patient is falling apart, or that he or she will require ongoing psychiatric help after the BMT.

Psychiatrists often help patients manage stress with sedatives and anti-depressant medications. Most BMT patients never before will have needed or used these medications. Short-term use of these drugs during the hospitalization is common, and does not mean the patient will develop a long-term drug dependency.

Sedatives and sleeping pills are particularly helpful in managing a very common problem experienced by BMT patients—insomnia. Deprived of sleep, a patient can quickly become exhausted, unfocused and extremely irritable, making it even harder to cope with daytime stresses. Medications are available to counteract insomnia; there's no need to put up with sleepless nights and the stress they produce.

BEING THERE FOR THE PATIENT

It's extremely important that family members be involved on a day-to-day basis with the patient's care. Often, the best thing that family members or friends can do for the patient is to just "be there."

Just having a loved one or friend close at hand can be very comforting. Don't feel you need to keep up a non-stop conversation during

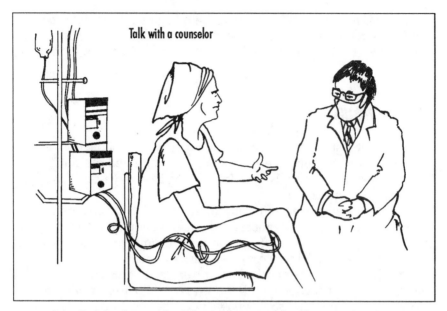

Talk with a counselor

your visit. Read, chat with the patient periodically, watch television—
share time as you would at home. It's your presence that counts most.

Throughout much of the hospitalization, the patient may be much
too weak to visit with guests or even accept phone calls. Nonetheless,
it's important for patients to know that family members, friends, and
co-workers are concerned about their progress and rooting for their
recovery. It can be very depressing for a patient to feel that he or she has
been forgotten by someone. Cards, handwritten notes, and words of
encouragement passed along through family members or friends can
mean a lot to a patient who feels isolated in a hospital room. Installing
an answering machine on the patient's phone is one way to let family
and friends communicate their well-wishes without requiring the
patient to engage in exhausting phone conversations.

Sometimes friends and acquaintances are afraid to "intrude" and
therefore do not call or write. If you're concerned, check first with a
family member; but more often than not your expression of concern will
boost the patient's spirits and help the recovery process. Other gestures
like donating platelets for the patient, helping with family household
chores, caring for the patient's children, providing an evening off for the
patient's support person, or filling in for the patient until she returns to
work will also be greatly appreciated.

Nights are an especially stressful time when patients feel most isolated and lonely. There are fewer distractions and fewer familiar faces
upon whom to rely for help. Alone in the dark, fears that normally grip
the patient during the day are intensified.

Many transplant facilities allow a support person to spend nights in the patient's room on a cot or daybed. Having a loved one present in the room at night greatly relieves patients' stress. If your transplant center does not routinely provide overnight accommodations for support persons,they may be willing to make special arrangements.

GETTING BACK TO NORMAL

The day of hospital discharge can be both exciting and frightening. On the one hand, patients are glad to leave the isolation of the hospital room behind them. On the other hand, losing the "safety net" of hospital personnel who've been available to support the patient's every medical need can be frightening.

The sights, sounds and smells of the world outside the hospital will assault the patient's senses. It's a very moving and exhausting experience when patients take the first step out of the hospital and start back on the road to a normal life.

During this period of recovery, patients desperately want to feel normal and be treated as such. They don't want pity. They want to be able to take care of themselves to the extent possible, and don't want to be singled out for special treatment unless absolutely necessary.

Family members, friends and co-workers sometimes have difficulty re-establishing their relationship with patients. Patients will look different. They may have lost weight, will have temporary hair loss, be wearing a face mask to protect against infection, or look physically drained. Because the patient will have been "out of circulation" for several weeks or months, he or she will not have shared as many experiences with family members or friends as usual. Visitors can feel awkward as they grope for an appropriate topic of conversation, and this awkwardness can discourage some people from calling or visiting.

In some cases, particularly with children, ignorance may make a person fearful of associating with the patient. One high school adolescent reported that, upon her return to school, the school corridors would literally clear out each time she appeared. The other children were afraid they might "catch it" and were uncomfortable interacting with a classmate they believed was about to die.

Friends and family members of patients can overcome some of this post-transplant awkwardness by not losing touch with patients while they're undergoing treatment. Sharing normal life experiences with the patient either during a visit, by a note, or with a phone call can help make the re-establishment of relationships post-transplant easier.

Children of adult transplant patients, as well as friends and classmates of children undergoing a transplant, should be prepared for the return of the patient, with the myths of "catching it" or the inevitability of the patient's death dispelled well in advance. This will not only ease the patient's stress, but relieve unspoken fears the children may have about their parent or friend.

Oftentimes friends will be unsure about how and when to re-establish a normal relationship with the patient, and will look for a cue from the patient before making a move. Some patients have found that asking friends to help with a small task such as picking up a prescription at the drug store, taking the patient's child to a school event, or returning a purchased item to a department store will "break the ice" and let

---

TIPS FOR SUPPORT PERSONS

A BMT is difficult, not only for the patient, but for support persons as well. This is especially true if the support person has ongoing family and/or job responsibilities. Here are a few tips that may help.

- Don't hesitate to ask other family members and friends for help in caring for the patient, your family, and **you** during the BMT. You'll need the help, and persons concerned about the patient's well-being will appreciate the opportunity to lend a hand.

- Be realistic about your limitations. Get enough sleep, eat properly, and take time off for yourself. You'll be a bigger help to the patient healthy and sane, than sick and overwhelmed.

- Be prepared for changes in the patient's behavior. The drugs and stress may cause the patient to become depressed or angry. He or she may say things that don't make sense or see things that aren't there. These changes are only temporary but can frighten support persons when they occur.

- At the same time, understand that your loved one needs you now more than ever before. Your help is not only welcome—it's absolutely essential.

- Don't be shy about tracking down the medical staff to get help or answers to your questions. You'll feel better knowing the doctors are aware of problems you've noted, and you're entitled to have all your questions answered fully.

- Finally, remember that as helpless as you may sometimes feel, the moral support you provide is often the best "medicine" the patient can get.

friends know that the patient is ready for their companionship.

Friends of transplant patients may help ease the transition back to normal life by inviting patients to accompany them to places or events that do not pose undue health risks. Despite the fact that the patients may need to wear a face mask when going on these excursions (which will make the experience less than perfect), their desire to get back into the normal flow of life may overcome their aversion to being conspicuous, and the invitation will be much appreciated.

During the recovery period, graft-versus-host disease (GVHD), a post-transplant side effect that affects many patients who undergo allogeneic transplants, can also be very stressful. GVHD is discussed at length in Chapter 9.

AND MANY MONTHS BEYOND

While some memories of the transplant experience dim with time, the trauma of the transplant will be remembered for many months, even years. It can take a very long time before a patient gets through a single day without reflecting on the transplant experience. Innocent remarks or events totally unrelated to the transplant may stir up unpleasant memories, leaving the patient shaken.

Many people who have been through the experience find it difficult to talk about, particularly with someone not intimately involved in the experience. They prefer to forget about the difficulties of the past, and go on with their lives.

Others want an outlet to talk about the experience. Support groups can be helpful for some patients, while others may prefer one-on-one discussions with counselors, other BMT patients, a family member or a friend.

Family members and friends of BMT patients often feel "shut out" by the patient who is unwilling to discuss her feelings with them. They must realize, however, that as much as the patient may love them and appreciate their concern, patients need to cope with the BMT experience at their own pace and in their own way. Unfortunately, patients seldom have enough emotional energy to help both themselves and their loved ones deal with the experience, no matter how grateful they are for their support.

A long-term, stressful side effect of the chemotherapy and/or radiation experienced by many BMT patients is infertility or sterility. Sperm banking, cryogenic embryo preservation, adoption, and assisted reproduction with donor sperm or ova are strategies some BMT patients are considering to cope with this problem. These options are discussed in more detail in Chapter 11.

Despite the emotional upheaval a transplant causes, life after transplant can be very special. Patients no longer take the future for granted, regardless of how promising their prognosis may be, and often enjoy each day of living more fully. As the months of survival turn into years, patients experience the added pleasure of being able once again to look forward to many more years of life.

On Saturday, June 15, 1991, we celebrated the 10th Anniversary of our Shands Hospital, University of Florida Bone Marrow Transplant Unit. It was a time of renewed acquaintances, and never was it clearer to us all that time heals. Many 'graduates' whom we had last seen struggling and weary from their time in the BMT unit were now returned to their shining, healthy selves. What an array! The laughter and tears flowed from all of us. Here is a poem dedicated to all who have faced this life challenge.

Unready Heroes

A lifetime of steady, schooling:
alphabet-rotes, number recital,
history's dates, cake-baking, fuse-fixing, slow-dancing,
how we are born and grow and age and die didn't ready you
for the naked facts
of our Consent Form.

A lifetime of educated modesty:
closing your bedroom door, covering your body,
segregating girls from boys,
separate facilities for men and women,
learned euphemisms for your body's functions -
didn't ready you for our free inspection
of your daily portapotti.

A lifetime of careless risk-taking:
climbing trees, jaywalking streets,
diving rock-pools, floating to sea,
driving fast cars, flying airplanes,
rash rollercoaster thrill-seeking -
didn't ready you for the chill reality
of this life-challenge.

A lifetime of practicing precaution:
sheltering from harm, not overdoing it,
running in the middle of the pack,
getting by with the least amount of effort,
okay grades without too much distinction didn't ready you
for our accolades
of this your hero's role.

John Graham-Pole, MD,
University of Florida,
Professor of Pediatrics

CHAPTER 7

When Your Child Needs a Bone Marrow Transplant

"It was like a whirlwind, a dream. One day our child was a normal 15-year-old boy who would live to be 80. The next day we were staring at blackboard diagrams about bone marrow transplants, and hearing doctors tell us our son might die. It wasn't real. We didn't understand. All we could do was hug each other and cry."

—Parents of BMT patient

Each year more than 2,000 children in the U.S. ranging in age from two months to 21 years undergo a BMT. They are battling diseases such as leukemia, aplastic anemia, immune deficiency disorders, inborn errors of metabolism and solid tumor cancers such a neuroblastoma. Depending on the type and stage of the disease, prior treatment, compatibility of donor marrow, and the child's general health, the odds of a successful BMT may be as high as 90 percent or less than 10 percent.

While pediatric BMTs are similar in many respects to adult BMTs, children undergoing BMTs and their parents have some concerns and needs that differ from adult BMT patients. This chapter will examine those issues, and share insights from parents, doctors, nurses, psychologists, social workers, and children about the experience.

DECIDING ON A BMT

Choosing whether or not to proceed with a bone marrow transplant is a difficult decision for children and parents alike. The odds of success must be weighed against the certainty that the BMT will be a lengthy, rigorous procedure. There is often no clear-cut "right" choice and parents and children can be frustrated at having to choose between equally unpleasant options.

Parents, particularly if their children are under age 14, have the authority and responsibility to make the final decision in most states.

Nonetheless, they know it is the child who must live with the conse-
quence of their decision and this can create internal turmoil. "I knew it
was a do or die situation," explained the mother of a 5-year-old boy
with aplastic anemia, "but I kept asking myself, 'Do I really have the
right to decide his life? I want to keep him with me as long as possible.
Am I deciding what's best for me or for him?'"

Most BMT centers and parents of former BMT patients strongly recommend involving the child in the decision-making process as much as
possible. Securing the child's cooperation and trust during the BMT is
imperative, and starts with a candid, caring explanation of the disease
and the BMT procedure.

Involving siblings in the early discussions about the child's disease
and treatment also helps unite the family and alleviate resentment other
children might feel toward the sick child and the attention he or she is
receiving. "We decided our 12-year-old son and his brother would be
told honestly about what was happening, and both would participate in
decision making as much as their age and maturity allowed," said one
mother whose son had a BMT for Hodgkin's disease. "Although this
placed a burden of maturity on both sons, they rose to meet it and our
family drew closer, frequently drawing support from each other."
Noted one psychologist, "Families who involve siblings in discussions
about the child's care and treatment often have fewer problems later on
with sibling jealousy or anger. Be completely honest with both the child
and siblings right from the start so there are no surprises down the road
and no feelings that they've been lied to."

GETTING INFORMATION

Finding and absorbing adequate information about BMTs prior to
making a final decision is not always easy. Most BMT centers will provide oral explanations of the procedure and explain the risks, potential
complications, and side effects, but not all have this information available in written form. This can make it difficult for parents to reflect on
the information they have been given, double check their understanding, and formulate new questions. It helps to have more than one adult
present during the explanations and to keep a journal of notes.

Sometimes parents receive conflicting information from their refer-
ring physician and the BMT team about the child's chances for survival,
side effects, or the urgency of a BMT. "The first conference with the
BMT team was the most depressing experience of my life—worse than
when my daughter was diagnosed," said the mother of an infant with
leukemia. "Our doctor never told us about the possible side effects. I

was terrified. I just wanted to grab my child and run."

Don't be shy about asking follow-up questions of the medical team, even if it's the 90th time the question has been asked. Keep asking until you understand and feel you have enough information upon which to base a decision. It is the medical team's job to make sure all questions are answered, no matter how long or how many repetitions it takes.

Many parents find it helpful to talk to parents of other children who have been through the procedure, particularly parents of a survivor. Your physician or BMT center, Candlelighters, or the BMT Newsletter may be able to put you in contact with such parents. Keep in mind, however, that despite their similarities, no two BMT experiences or centers will be exactly alike.

Children's questions and concerns about the BMT vary according to their age. Younger children focus on immediate problems like how much it will hurt, whether they will be separated from their parents, when they can return to school, when their hair will grow back, whether or not they'll vomit a lot, and whether they will have to have chemotherapy after the BMT. After acquiring a basic understanding of the procedure, younger children tend to rely on their parents to decide what's best.

Teens, on the other hand, take a much more active role in the decision-making process and, by law, must give their consent to the procedure in most states. They tend to be very concerned about their self image and worry about losing their hair, gaining weight from steroids, etc. They're concerned about fitting in with their peers once the BMT is over and returning to a normal school life.

The possibility of infertility post-transplant can be distressing for an adolescent. Sexual identity and activity are important to teens and they may erroneously believe that infertility means they'll be unable to have an active sex life. The notion of infertility can be particularly distressing if discussions of "family" or "parenting" have always been narrowed to include only a traditional, biological family, as opposed to a family with adopted children or children conceived with the help of medically assisted reproduction techniques. While sperm banking for young males is a possibility, teens are sometimes too embarrassed to discuss or attempt this option.

Parents typically focus on longer term questions such as the risk of relapse, problems of non-engraftment, graft-versus-host disease, and how long after transplant the child will remain susceptible to infection. Parents also are usually distressed over the prospect of post-transplant infertility. Some are disappointed that they may not have grandchildren, ignoring the possibility that the child might build a family through adoption or medically assisted reproduction if infertility does occur. Parents of children who are very young at the time of the BMT worry about how best to prepare their child for a discussion of this problem in the future, when to raise the issue, what to say, and what reaction to expect.

"Discussing infertility with very young children who are still in the process of distinguishing between boys and girls and establishing their own gender can hurt more than help, especially if the issue is being raised in the midst of a medical crisis like a BMT," stated one psychologist. "The age of 9 or 10 is a good time to begin talking about it. It's helpful to normalize the situation, to let them know that many adults (one in six) are infertile and to distinguish between child-bearing and child-rearing. As they reach puberty, it will become more of an issue and distinguishing between infertility and having a normal sex life will be important. This is not an issue that can be dealt with in one marathon session and then ignored. Children will have questions and feelings about it for a long time and should be encouraged to talk about them."

Occasionally there is disagreement between parents and children about whether or not to proceed with a BMT. These cases often involve a child for whom a BMT offers only a small chance of long term survival and/or who is distressed at the prospect of infertility. Resolving these conflicts can be difficult but is essential. "Listen to each other carefully," advised one BMT nurse coordinator "and respect the child's concerns as well as your own."

Disagreements between parents about the wisdom of proceeding with a BMT are also not unusual. "At first I was totally against it because the chance of success seemed so low," said one infant's mother. "Even the doctors had conflicting opinions. I was really torn. I finally decided that if we found a matching bone marrow donor, the BMT was meant to be. We did, and my daughter is now doing fine."

"We had just gotten our son back to the point where he seemed happy and healthy and now they were proposing a BMT," said another mother. "I kept thinking, 'Why take him back to ground zero? Why can't we leave him alone?'"

PREPARING FOR THE TRANSPLANT

Once the decision to proceed with the BMT has been made, numerous preparations begin. The child who will undergo the procedure, the siblings, parents and members of the extended family must all be prepared for the physically and emotionally difficult times that lie ahead. Parents, particularly those with other children, may feel pulled in several directions, trying to help the sick child, their spouse, and their other children cope with the experience. Other family members and friends can best help by listening to parents about what they want and need during this period of time, responding to those requests, and respecting the parents' right to make decisions even if they themselves would decide things differently.

For the child undergoing the BMT, this will usually be the first life experience with such a rigorous, challenging, situation and the intense emotions it involves. Younger children may fear that they themselves are to blame for the disease and treatment, that they were somehow naughty and are being punished. Young siblings may also fear that they caused the problem, e.g.. they got angry with the sick child and said "I wish you'd get sick and die" and now it is coming to pass.

It is important that children of all ages be encouraged to discuss their feelings openly so their concerns can be addressed. Find out what your child is thinking. Don't assume that if he or she doesn't talk about the illness or BMT, there's no problem. Sometimes concerns and anxieties will be expressed through behavioral changes rather than verbally, e.g.. nightmares, belligerence, depression, etc. It is important for parents to help children understand that they did not cause the disease and that the treatment is not a punishment but the best way to try and make the disease go away. Parents should let their children know that they understand they are unhappy, frightened and confused and that the parents share their unhappiness, but that together they will work hard to help the child get well again.

Sometimes children will more openly discuss their feelings with someone other than their parents. This is particularly true of pre-adolescents and adolescents who are fearful of hurting their parents' feelings or causing them distress. Adolescents who are coping with typical teen desires for independence may be especially reluctant to "let down their guard" in the presence of parents. While parents may resent or be hurt by this fact, it is important that children be able to discuss their feelings when they are ready to do so with whomever they feel most comfortable. Parents can seek the help of nurses, psychologists or other counselors to encourage the child to open up if the child will not do so in their presence.

Children about to undergo a BMT should be thoroughly familiar with the hospital, the people with whom they will come in contact, and the equipment that will be used during the procedure. Children should be shown unfamiliar devices like the catheters and IV poles and given simple, clear explanations about what these devices do, why they are needed, and what it will feel like when they are used. Allowing children to handle the hospital equipment and try out the procedures on dolls before they enter the hospital often helps them get comfortable with the equipment, allows them to ask questions, and reduces their fear when it is eventually used during treatment.

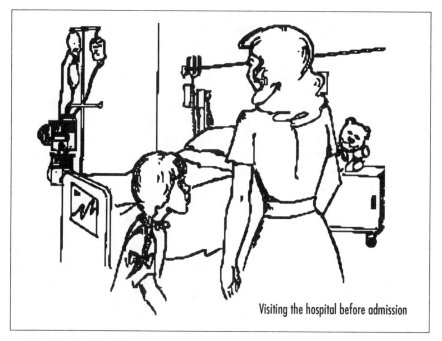

Visiting the hospital before admission

SIBLINGS' CONCERNS

Bringing siblings to the hospital and showing them where their brother or sister will spend the next several weeks is a good idea. They will feel less left out as preparations for the BMT begin and will have a better sense of where their sibling will be and what will be done to their sibling.

Often siblings must be left in the care of friends or relatives while the child is in the hospital. This may involve removing the siblings from their home and normal routines. Young children may view this forced separation from their parents as a punishment. It is important that siblings know that the parent doesn't want this separation, that it will be temporary, and why it is not possible for the child to stay with the parent. Creating a "home away from home" environment with routines of play, study, eating, etc. as similar to the child's normal home routine as possible helps. Setting up a plan of routine contact between the parents and siblings will lessen the feeling that they are being ignored or that they aren't loved as much as the sick child. "Every day I would call my daughter and write her a note," said one parent whose daughter stayed with grandparents during her brother's BMT. "When I wrote, I would tell her what was happening with her brother, but when I called, I made sure we talked about her."

If siblings stay with their parents during the hospitalization, the professional staff can be helpful in talking with them and addressing their concerns. Some centers have special programs designed to help siblings through the experience.

THE SIBLING DONOR

Often so much time and energy is focused on the child to be transplanted that the needs and concerns of a sibling who is to be a marrow donor are underestimated. For these children, the medical procedure they're about to undergo is no less daunting or frightening than that awaiting their brother or sister. They too need careful preparation to make sure their questions and concerns are addressed and they need to feel that their parents are just as concerned about them as they are about the child about to receive the BMT. Members of the extended family and friends should also be made aware of the needs of the donor as well as the child who is ill. "Friends kept calling and asking how my son was doing," said one parent. "I told them he was fine, it was my daughter the donor who was hurting and needed their attention right now."

Parents, relatives, friends, or members of the BMT team sometimes try to secure a sibling donor's cooperation or attempt to bolster his ego by stressing that his marrow will save the sick child's life. Rather than make the donor feel important, however, this kind of talk can impose a terrible sense of personal responsibility on the child for the success or failure of the BMT, a situation that is totally out of his control. If the transplanted child's blood counts do not progress well, if complications arise, or if the child eventually dies, the sibling may suffer tremendous guilt and depression. Even if explicit statements to this effect are not made to a child donor, these feelings of responsibility may nonetheless exist and should be addressed.

WAITING FOR THE TRANSPLANT

Once preparations for the BMT have been finalized, families can feel "at sea." Being anxious about the BMT, re-thinking the wisdom of proceeding with the transplant, and continually working through their own fears as well as their children's concerns during this waiting period can be very stressful. Providing parents and children an opportunity to talk about their concerns, or engaging them in a special outing or event to help distract their attention from the problem for a few hours is a helpful service that friends and extended family members can give.

It is not unusual for stresses that previously existed in a home or marriage to be heightened during this time. Plans for a separation or divorce may get put on hold as a result of the planned BMT, with tensions between marital partners increasing. Substance abuse problems may become acute as a result of the added stress. Don't be embarrassed to seek help for these problems—you won't be the first person to do so. In general, it is best to make as few changes as possible in the home routine and keep lines of communication open during this difficult time.

LIFE DURING TRANSPLANT

Although a BMT is anything but routine, it is important to maintain as much of the child's normal home routine as possible while in the hospital. Bringing along favorite clothes, pictures, toys, etc. helps maintain a sense of normalcy. Arranging for calls, letters and/or visits from the child's classmates, favorite teacher, church members, or from a hometown doctor with whom the child feels comfortable can also help. Some families make videos of families and friends that the child can view while in the hospital.

Despite everyone's best efforts, the hospitalization will be a very stressful time for child and parents alike. Children will be inundated with tests, medications and daily medical procedures. Children of all ages, and teens in particular, feel overwhelmed by all the rules and "bosses," and can become angry over the loss of personal control. This manifests itself in several ways.

Some become angry or belligerent, refusing to cooperate with parents and/or the medical staff. Others will cry for no apparent reason and be unable to explain what is making them sad. A child may refuse to eat or play. Still others may become depressed, listless or exhibit regressive or babyish behavior e.g.. they'll be incapable of performing tasks they were previously able to do on their own. Parents usually bear the brunt of the behavioral changes.

"Children spend a whole lot of time and energy growing up, seizing control over their life, and becoming more independent," explained one psychologist. "When they undergo a BMT, they lose that independence and control, and that can make them angry or depressed."

"Children don't feel the same urgency about routine medical procedures as parents do," noted a BMT nurse. "It's important to talk with children and let them know that you know it's hard, and to let them know that feeling angry is normal and OK."

"I never said to my son 'don't cry,'" said one mother. "I encouraged him to talk about what was bothering him and to let it all out. If he really rebelled against doing something like mouth care, I wouldn't insist it be done that moment. We'd talk about it and usually it would get done without a fight five minutes later. Sometimes I'd suggest we do it a few minutes before the nurse came in so that he could feel like it was his decision and not her order that made it happen. He liked that feeling of control."

"Children are as concerned about protecting their body and having control over their personal life as adults," explained a child therapist. "Treat them as persons. Don't violate their bodies without asking permission. Give them the opportunity to say 'no' or to make choices regarding their care or daily activities whenever it's possible for you to honor their decision."

Setting up and sticking to a daily routine in the hospital is important for children. Ideally, the routine should include some "safe" time for the child each day in which no unpleasant tests, medications, or staff intervention occurs. At one center, a child's parents created a "safe area" for the child in the room by bringing in a free-standing tent. When the child needed time alone, she would go into the tent to play.

Preparing children immediately in advance of each new medication or medical procedure is very important. Children need to know what

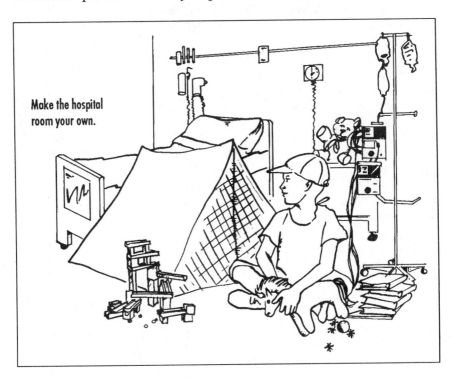

Make the hospital room your own.

will be done, what the equipment will look like, and how they will feel during the procedure. Often a child's imagination can conjure up a more terrifying picture of the procedure than is actually the case. Younger children can misunderstand language used to describe the procedure and can become unnecessarily frightened. They may imagine a "shot" for example to be a gunshot rather than a needle pricking their arm. Children should be told about the medication or procedure far enough in advance to allow them to work through questions, but not so far in advance that they will have time to brood about it.

Advance explanation is even required before the administration of drugs designed to ease pain or sedate the child. "The first time my child was given Demerol (a pain medication) he became almost violent. He wasn't prepared for the feeling of grogginess and it frightened him. After that, I always made sure he knew in advance how the drugs would make him feel," reported one mother.

Boredom in the hospital can be a big issue for children. Bringing favorite toys, games, etc. from home helps to ease the boredom. Planning diversions and activities for teens is especially important. "My son was 15-years-old in a children's hospital. Although they had lots of activities planned, they were usually geared toward younger kids, not teens," noted one parent.

The time in the hospital is difficult for parents as well. It's hard to watch your child undergo difficult medical procedures, particularly when you have so little control over her care. "They kept saying that 'being there' for my child was important," said one mother,"but it never felt like I was doing enough." Said another, "I worried constantly because my child was too little to talk to us and tell us if he hurt."

Parents can be important advocates for their children, particularly when it comes to securing pain relief or minimizing the discomfort associated with medical procedures. Some BMT centers, for example, usually administer sedatives or other pain control medications to children in advance of bone marrow aspirates (a medical procedure that can be very uncomfortable) while others do not. Don't hesitate to ask for pain medication if your child has difficulty with a procedure and don't feel intimidated if the medical staff initially resists your request without providing a good reason.

It is important for parents to pace themselves during this time so that they don't become exhausted or ill. Taking a few minutes or hours off while social workers or visitors spend time with the child can be helpful. Some parents find that spending the night away from the hospital enables them to get a good night's rest and better cope with the next day's stresses. For other parents, remaining with the child overnight is less stressful and preferable.

Children are very perceptive about their parents' feelings, and can be frightened when they detect sadness or stress in their parents. Some children may feel guilty, thinking they caused their parents' sadness, and a desire to protect their parents can be a stumbling block to speaking frankly about their own concerns. Acknowledging that the hospitalization is scary for everyone involved and that everyone will work through the experience is important.

"Every day my son would say 'I love you, thank you for being here with me. It makes it easier when I'm not feeling good,'" said the mother of a fifth-grader. "They know it's just as hard for you as it is for them."

GOING HOME

Going home—the day that everyone waits for—can be a bittersweet experience. Although the hospitalization has ended, the recovery period is far from over. Medications must be administered several times daily, central lines (the catheter or flexible tubing through which blood samples are drawn and medications and transfusions are administered) must be cleaned, and several visits per week must be made to the outpatient clinic to monitor the child's progress. Parents will be "on pins and needles" watching for signs of infection or other complications. It is not uncommon for problems to develop that require the child to be readmitted to the hospital for a short time and this can be alarming for parents and children alike.

"Picking up the pieces is not easy," said one mother. "For months I felt like I was on autopilot. I forgot how to sleep and constantly felt like I was dragging. There didn't seem to be enough hours in the day or energy in me to take care of everyone's needs. After ten months I wondered 'when will this be over?'"

Frequently, friends and extended family fail to understand that the trauma continues long after a child returns home. "They think that once you walk out the door of the hospital, everything is behind you, that you should pick up life where you left off. It just doesn't work that way," said several parents. "It would really drive me crazy when people would say 'you must feel so lucky' or 'you must be so grateful' when I was feeling anything but lucky," said another parent. "While I was grateful to have witnessed a miracle, I was still really angry that our family had to go through all this. I kept wondering 'why us? What did we do to deserve this?'"

The reunion of the siblings with the parent who spent time at the hospital with the BMT child is not always a smooth one. "At first my 3-year-old refused to talk to me," said one mother. Said another, "My daughter was left in my husband's care at home during my son's BMT.

She talked with my husband and treated him like her parent, but closed up to me. That hurt a lot. We found a therapist who helped us understand her fears and resentments, and work through them."

Siblings often feel resentful or jealous of the extra attention the child undergoing the BMT continues to receive after returning home. They may express a desire to be sick so their mother will pay more attention to them. They can resent the fact that different rules apply to them than to the BMT child. Some parents have found that involving the sibling in the routine caregiving can make them feel needed and important. Setting aside time for the parent and sibling to do something special together also helps.

"I told visitors who planned to bring my son a gift to bring one for his sister as well, or bring nothing at all," said a parent. "It was hard for her to see her brother get all the attention. She felt shut out."

The child undergoing a BMT often senses the sadness siblings feel over the lack of attention shown them. Said one little boy to his sister, "I'm sorry I'm so lazy right now and mom's doing everything for me. As soon as I feel better you can have mommy for awhile."

Behavioral problems with the child undergoing a BMT are not uncommon after transplant. "Parents get set up to be in an awkward position when they return home," said one nurse. "While in the hospital, the child will usually get lots of cards, gifts, balloons and attention and may expect it to continue at home. If the level of attention diminishes, the child may become angry and resentful."

Both the child undergoing a BMT and siblings may become very anxious over symptoms of a common cold or other minor discomforts after the BMT. Said one mother, "I went to my son's room one night when I heard him sniffling. 'This feels so familiar,' he said. 'I always used to get sick at night and you'd have to take me to the hospital.' When I assured him that he would be OK he said, 'That sounds familiar too.'"

"Our daughter was afraid to get sick after her brother's BMT," said another parent. "When she got the flu last week it was the first time that she was the sick one rather than her brother. He hovered over her, rubbing her back, bringing her something to drink, trying to soothe her. They were both very concerned."

"Don't ignore or trivialize a sibling's complaints of illness," advised a BMT nurse. "Show them you are as concerned about their well-being as you are about the BMT child. Call the doctor even if you think it is something minor. It can help put their mind at ease."

"Don't assume siblings' complaints of illness are a deliberate ploy to get attention," advised a psychologist. "Children often mimic symptoms of the illness unconsciously, and truly believe they are ill."

Certain post-transplant events that parents view as milestones can unexpectedly be very traumatic for the child. A 2-year old, for example, became very upset when his central line was removed. "We thought he'd be happy to get rid of it. Instead, he became very upset—it was like part of his body was being removed," said one mom.

Returning to school is a milestone that children are often encouraged to look forward to, but it too can be a tremendous letdown. They may find their classmates are not awaiting their return with baited breath, that their friends have moved on to new interests and activities without them, or that other children are fearful of associating with a child that has been sick and may now look different. "It helps to prepare classmates in advance for the child's return," advises a social worker. "A nurse, doctor or social worker can visit the school, explain what has happened to the child, and answer questions." Even with advance preparation, however, the child undergoing a BMT sometimes finds it difficult to fit back in.

Despite the difficulties, the BMT experience often brings families closer together. "My children still squabble a lot, but they're very concerned and protective of each other as well," said one parent." "It was rough while we went through it, but the good times have come now," said another mother. "My son made it, he's healthy, and we all appreciate what it means to be alive."

CHAPTER 8

Infections

The air we breathe, the food we eat, the hands we shake, the items we touch—everything we contact in daily life is a potential source of bacteria, viruses or fungi that can cause infection. For a normal, healthy individual these daily encounters with sources of infection are not a major problem. The body and its immune system work to protect the body from infections or efficiently destroy them if they enter the body.

For BMT patients, however, it's a different story. The chemotherapy and/or radiation administered prior to a BMT cannot distinguish between cancerous and normal cells, and thus attacks not only the cancer or diseased bone marrow, but disrupts the patient's immune system as well. Skin and mucous membranes, the body's first line of defense against infection, may be damaged. White blood cells, part of the body's internal defense team, are destroyed. Special proteins called "antibodies" that normally help destroy bacteria and viruses such as measles or chicken pox are depleted. Until the transplanted bone marrow engrafts and produces new white blood cells, BMT patients are extremely vulnerable to infections that in some cases can be life threatening.

The first two to four weeks after the transplant is a particularly critical time as the transplanted bone marrow migrates to the cavities of the large bones and begins producing new white blood cells. Although the risk of infection steadily declines once the transplanted marrow begins producing new white blood cells, most patients' immune systems remain "compromised" (not functioning at 100 percent efficiency) for six months to a year after the transplant, and often longer for patients with graft-versus-host disease.

During the first month post-BMT, the risk of infection is the same for both autologous and allogeneic BMT patients. Thereafter, allogeneic BMT patients, especially those with GVHD, are more likely to develop infections than autologous BMT patients. GVHD prolongs the period of time during which the immune system is compromised and the patient remains susceptible to infection.

Although post-transplant infections are a serious cause for concern, great strides have been made over the past ten years to better manage and prevent infections, and deaths from infections have declined significantly.

FIGHTING INFECTION—THE IMMUNE SYSTEM

The immune system is the body's defense network against infection and disease. Many organs, tissues, cells, and proteins make up the immune system, each with a specific role to play in the body's defense.

Skin and the mucous membranes lining the mouth and nose provide the body's first line of defense against invading organisms and foreign substances, and repel millions of harmful organisms daily. If a cut occurs, infectious organisms can invade the body, causing white blood cells or "leukocytes" to spring into action.

Leukocytes patrol the body via the bloodstream or the lymph system and take up residence in tissues, seeking out and destroying foreign matter that invades the body. (The lymph system, which transports cells and waste products of the immune system, is a network of vessels running alongside the bloodstream.)

Leukocytes evolve from "stem cells," which are produced in the bone marrow. Those that play a key role in protecting the body against infection, disease, and other foreign substances are lymphocytes, macrophages, monocytes, neutrophils, and natural killer cells.

Lymphocytes

There are two kinds of lymphocytes: "T-cells" and "B-cells." T-cells recognize foreign particles in the body, orchestrate their destruction, and shut down the "immune system response" or attack once the foreign matter has been destroyed.

Viruses, parasites and bacteria that invade the body are composed of cells. On the surface of each cell are genetic markers called "antigens." The immune system knows which antigens belong in a person's body and which do not. When "helper" T-cells spot a foreign antigen in the body, they stimulate the production of "killer" T-cells, which engulf and destroy the invading cell. "Suppressor" T-cells shut down the immune system attack once the foreign cell is destroyed.

Helper T-cells can also order the second type of lymphocytes—B-cells—into action. Helper T-cells point out foreign antigens to the B-cells which, in turn, manufacture a Y-shaped protein called an "immunoglobulin" or "antibody." The antibody zeroes in on the antigen and attaches to the surface of the invading cell. The antibody then summons the "complement system"—a group of proteins circulating in the bloodstream—to surround the cell and dissolve a hole in it. This process is called cell lysis. When the dissolution is completed, other white blood cells clean up the remains of the destroyed cell, and suppressor T-cells shut down the B-cell activity.

Over the course of a lifetime, millions of antibodies are produced by B-cells. Once an antibody has been produced, it circulates through the body for many years, making the body "immune" to further attacks by that particular antigen.

Other Leukocytes

Monocytes, macrophages, and neutrophils are often referred to collectively as "phagocytes." These scavenger cells engulf and destroy some invading particles, and clean up the remains of others that have been destroyed by T-cells or B-cells. Natural killer cells are another type of leukocyte that can recognize and destroy some tumor cells.

To function properly, the immune system needs all types of white blood cells in sufficient quantity and in the proper ratio in the bloodstream. If the bone marrow, which produces white blood cells, malfunctions or is destroyed, the body can no longer fight off serious and sometimes fatal infections.

BACTERIAL INFECTIONS

Bacteria are microscopic organisms that invade tissues and multiply rapidly. Bacteria can cause infections anywhere in the body, and are the usual cause of ear and sinus infections, as well as bronchitis.

Bacteria secrete poisonous chemicals called "toxins" that interfere with normal organ functions. Toxins can, among other things, cause shock or low blood pressure that can lead to death if insufficient oxygen is provided to the heart or brain.

Bacteria can also disrupt normal organ functions by their sheer number. Some pneumonias, for example, are caused by rapidly multiplying bacteria which fill up the spaces in lungs where air is normally absorbed into the body.

Bacterial infections are most common during the first two to four weeks following a BMT, occurring in 50 percent of patients. The chemotherapy and/or radiation administered prior to the transplant impair a patient's ability to fight bacterial infections in three ways.

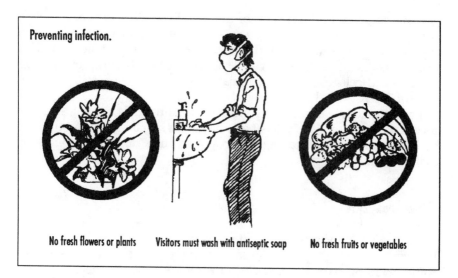

Preventing infection.

No fresh flowers or plants   Visitors must wash with antiseptic soap   No fresh fruits or vegetables

First, the skin and mucous membrane barriers which normally prevent bacteria from entering the body are damaged. Second, neutrophils—the white blood cells responsible for fighting bacteria—are destroyed, making patients "neutropenic." Third, antibodies that once made the patient immune to certain bacterial infections are depleted.

Post-BMT bacterial infections occur most often in intestines, on the skin (especially around Hickman catheters or the central line), and in the mouth. They also occasionally occur in the bladder and can cause pneumonia in the lungs.

To combat bacterial infections, large doses of antibiotics such as aminoglycosides, penicillins, cephalosporins or vancomycin are usually administered during the first few weeks post-transplant if the patient's temperature rises above 101°. Patients bathe or shower daily to remove bacteria from their skin. Careful oral hygiene to destroy bacteria in the mouth is generally required. Soft toothbrushes or sponges are used to cleanse the gums and teeth so that cuts through which bacteria, fungi and viruses may enter can be avoided.

Hospital staff and visitors carefully wash their hands with antiseptic soap prior to touching the patient (since hands are a primary carrier of infectious agents), and may also wear protective masks, gowns or gloves while in the patient's room. Flowers and plants (both live and dried) which can harbor harmful bacteria or fungi are not permitted in the room while the patient is neutropenic. Similarly, fresh fruits and vegetables are eliminated from the patient's diet until the immune system begins functioning properly.

When detected promptly and treated with antibiotics, bacterial infections are usually not fatal.

FUNGAL INFECTIONS

Fungi are primitive life forms that we encounter daily. Bread mold is an example of a common fungus. Most are harmless and some, such as the fungus called Candida, normally reside inside our bodies.

Fungal infections are common in BMT patients during the first three months post-transplant, particularly among allogeneic BMT patients with graft-versus-host disease. Ironically, while the widespread use of antibiotics post-transplant has successfully reduced the incidence of harmful bacterial infections, these antibiotics may also destroy beneficial bacteria in the body that keep fungi in check.

Fungal infections are very difficult to detect and treat. Candida and Aspergillus infections are the most common post-transplant fungal infections.

Candida fungi live in the intestines, mouth and vagina and are normally kept in check by bacteria. When bacteria are destroyed by antibiotics, however, the fungus can multiply and spread, infecting many parts of the body.

Aspergillus infections occur most often in the sinus passages or lungs, and can cause pneumonia. Aspergillus fungi are frequently found around construction sites or where buildings are being remodeled.

At some BMT centers, special air-filtering equipment is installed in patients' rooms to remove fungi from the air. Eliminating fresh plants, fruits and vegetables from the patient's environment also reduces the risk of fungal infections.

Amphotericin B, an anti-fungal medication, is usually given to patients who have continuous fevers after taking antibiotics in an attempt to control the development of fungal infections. Research is underway for other anti-fungal treatments since amphotericin B may be toxic and can interfere with the effectiveness of drugs given to control

---

USUAL CAUSES OF INFECTION POST-TRANSPLANT

MONTH 1
bacteria
fungi
herpes simplex virus

MONTHS 2-3
cytomegalovirus*
other viruses*
bacteria*
fungi*

MONTHS 4-12
varicella zoster virus*
bacteria*
fungi*

More common following allogeneic BMTs than autologous BMTs, particularly in patients with graft-versus-host disease.

graft-versus-host disease. A drug called fluconazole has been shown to be effective in treating Candida infections in clinical trials and is now often used as a preventive medication.

Historically, Aspergillus infections have been difficult to treat and infected patients have often died. New techniques used to diagnose Aspergillus infections earlier, as well as the use of amphotericin B have helped reduce the number of deaths from Aspergillus infections.

VIRAL INFECTIONS

Viruses are tiny parasites, smaller than bacteria, that are not self-sufficient. They must invade other organisms, such as human cells, in order to survive and multiply. Viruses tinker with the genetic machinery of the "host" cell, turning it into a factory for the production of more of the virus. The virus eventually destroys or cripples the host cell and moves on to neighboring cells to continue its reproduction and destruction.

Infections caused by viruses are very difficult to treat. Because few effective anti-viral medications are available, healthy individuals rely on T-cells and antibodies produced by B-cells to keep invading viruses in check. Several anti-viral agents such as acyclovir and ganciclovir are useful, but the number of viruses they effectively treat is small.

Viral infections following a BMT can occur either as a result of exposure to a new virus or reactivation of an old virus dormant in the patient's body. The chemotherapy and/or radiation administered to the patient prior to the transplant destroys T-cells and depletes antibodies responsible for keeping viruses in check.

Viral infections are most common during the first 12 months following a BMT, but may occur as late as two years post-transplant. Those most commonly seen in BMT patients are caused by the herpes simplex virus (HSV), cytomegalovirus (CMV), and varicella zoster virus (VZV).

Herpes Simplex

Herpes simplex infections are caused by two separate viruses: Herpes 1 and Herpes 2. "Oral herpes" (the Herpes 1 virus) causes painful fever blisters around and in the mouth. "Genital herpes" (the Herpes 2 virus) causes painful blisters on the genitalia and/or rectum.

An estimated 70 percent of Americans are exposed to the Herpes 1 virus, usually during childhood. The virus is highly contagious and is usually transmitted through contact with persons having active herpes sores on their mouths. Herpes 2, on the other hand, is usually transmitted through sexual intercourse with an infected partner.

Herpes infections often recur after the initial episode. The virus can lay dormant in the body for many years, flaring up at predictable or unpredictable intervals. Even if a person does not recall having had an active case of herpes, the virus may nonetheless be present in the body.

Herpes infections usually occur during the first month following a BMT. They're almost always caused by a herpes virus present in the body prior to the transplant.

In addition to the usual mouth sores associated with a Herpes 1 infection, skin lesions are sometimes associated with a Herpes 1 infection in BMT patients. In rare cases, a Herpes 1 infection can occur in the brain.

Herpes simplex is one of the viruses that responds well to treatment with anti-viral agents. Acyclovir taken orally or administered intravenously is the usual treatment. Most centers now administer prophylactic (preventive) doses of acyclovir, which has greatly reduced the incidence of post-transplant herpes infections.

Cytomegalovirus (CMV)

CMV or cytomegalovirus is a common cause of infection in BMT patients. Approximately 30 percent of patients undergoing a BMT develop a CMV infection, usually during the second or third month following the transplant.

CMV infections can develop in several different organs including the liver, colon, eye, and lungs. Although all CMV infections are cause for concern, CMV pneumonia is particularly worrisome because it's usually fatal. A CMV infection in the intestines is often fatal as well.

Approximately half the general population is exposed to CMV during their lifetime, particularly urban dwellers. Doctors can test a patient's blood prior to transplant to determine whether or not CMV is present in their body. If it is not, the patient is "CMV-negative" and care is taken to prevent exposure to CMV before, during and after the transplant. If possible, a CMV-negative bone marrow donor is used. Blood products given to patients are often screened to ensure they are CMV-negative before being infused into patients. Alternatively, some BMT centers administer intravenous immunoglobulin when CMV-negative blood products are not available.

Patients who test positive for CMV prior to transplant are twice as likely to develop a CMV infection post-transplant than those who test negative. Patients undergoing an allogeneic BMT are more likely to develop a CMV infection than autologous BMT patients, particularly if they receive bone marrow from a mismatched donor.

Some two to four percent of autologous BMT patients, and approximately 10 to 20 percent of allogeneic BMT patients develop CMV pneumonia. The risk of developing CMV pneumonia increases with age and among patients with graft-versus-host disease.

Recent studies suggest that a new drug called ganciclovir used in combination with intravenous immunoglobulin can effectively treat CMV pneumonia. Other studies are underway to determine whether ganciclovir is an effective preventive therapy for CMV infections.

Varicella Zoster Virus

Varicella Zoster virus (VZV) is sometimes referred to as "shingles" or "herpes zoster." It is the same virus that causes chicken pox. Twenty to 40 percent of BMT patients develop a VZV infection during the first year post-transplant, usually after the third month. VZV infections occur most frequently in allogeneic BMT patients with graft-versus-host disease, but are common among autologous BMT patients as well.

VZV infections manifest themselves in one of two ways. The first involves an itching, blistering skin rash extending along any one of the body's nerve branches. The nerve endings under the skin at the site of the rash are infected and can cause great pain.

The second involves the ophthalmic nerve or nerve to the eye. A painful rash may occur along the nerve path on the forehead and eyelids and, if not treated promptly, can damage the eye.

VZV infections are usually treated with acyclovir intravenously over a seven-day period. They are quite contagious, and a hospital stay is usually required for treatment. While in the hospital, medications such as Tylenol, codeine or morphine may be administered to control pain. Early treatment can reduce the pain associated with VZV infections. VZV infections are not fatal if treated promptly.

A VZV infection can occur more than once post-transplant. The itching and/or pain associated with a VZV infection can continue long after all clinical signs of the disease disappear.

Acyclovir given to prevent herpes and CMV infections can also be effective in the prevention of VZV infections. Since VZV infections are highly contagious, patients who have never had chicken pox or who've had a negative blood test for VZV should avoid people with chicken pox or VZV infections for the first year following a BMT.

Other Viruses

Other viruses such as adenovirus, papovavirus, Epstein-Barr virus

---

PREVENTING INFECTIONS

There are several steps BMT patients can take to minimize the risk of infections:

- Avoid crowds and people with infections.

- Wear a face mask when in crowds.

- Avoid persons recently inoculated with live viruses such as chicken pox.

- Don't change diapers of a baby who's recently been inoculated.

- Wash your hands frequently, especially before handling food.

- Don't swim in public pools or lakes for at least a year post-transplant.

- Minimize your exposure to animals, particularly barnyard animals. Don't handle animal feces.

- Avoid construction sites and home remodeling while you're still susceptible to infection.

- Check with your doctor before being inoculated with live vaccines, e.g. the measles vaccine.

- At the first sign of fever or infection, call your physician. Infections are most easily treated when caught early. Infections you used to ignore or "tough out" can be serious problems post-transplant.

(EBV), respiratory syncitial virus (RSV), and human papilloma virus (HPV) can also create problems post-transplant, although the incidence of these infections is quite low.

Adenovirus and RSV infections can cause fatal pneumonia. Adenovirus can also cause infections in the kidneys or gastrointestinal tract and bleeding in the urine. In rare cases, the Epstein-Barr virus infects the lymph system of allogeneic BMT patients, creating a lymphoma-like condition which is often fatal.

The likelihood of developing these viral infections can be greatly reduced by limiting contact with the public post-transplant, wearing face masks, and meticulous hand washing.

PROTOZOA

Protozoa are single cell parasites that feed on organisms such as human cells to survive. T-cells provide the primary defense against protozoan infections. Although infections from protozoa are less common than bacterial or viral infections, they can pose serious problems for BMT patients who are T-cell deficient.

One protozoan called Pneumocystis carinii often lurks harmlessly in the trachea or windpipe of healthy human beings. When a person's immune system becomes suppressed, however, this protozoan may enter the lungs and grow into tiny cysts which cause pneumonia. Bactrim or Septra and pentamidine are highly effective in preventing and treating Pneumocystis carinii pneumonia.

Another infection called toxoplasmosis occasionally develops in patients post-BMT. Toxoplasmosis is caused by a protozoan called Toxoplasma gondii, which is often transmitted in the feces of cats. Toxoplasmosis may infect the brain, eyes, muscles, liver and/or lungs. A painful, inflamed retina in the eye is a common manifestation of the disease, which, without prompt treatment can result in damage to the eye. With early diagnosis and proper treatment, toxoplasmosis is seldom fatal.

DON'T TAKE CHANCES

It's tempting to throw caution to the wind after a BMT and ignore the threat of infections. Keep in mind, however, that bacteria, viruses and fungi that are harmless to most people can cause very serious and sometimes fatal infections in BMT patients whose immune systems are not fully recovered post-transplant. *Don't take chances.*

Avoiding sources of infection post-BMT can be inconvenient and frustrating, but a few months of caution are well worth saving your life.

CHAPTER 9

Graft-versus-host Disease

Graft-versus-host disease is a frequent complication of allogeneic BMTs. In GVHD, the donor's bone marrow attacks the patient's organs and tissues, impairing their ability to function, and increasing the patient's susceptibility to infection.

Approximately 50 percent of patients undergoing an allogeneic BMT with a related HLA-matched donor develop GVHD. Fortunately, the majority of cases are mild. GVHD is not a complication of autologous BMTs.

GVHD is often discussed as if it were a single disease. It is, in fact, two diseases: acute GVHD and chronic GVHD. Patients may develop one, both or neither. Acute and chronic GVHD differ in their symptoms, clinical signs and time of onset. (Clinical signs are the results of physical exams, x-rays or lab tests that confirm the existence and extent of a disease.)

GVHD can be a temporary inconvenience or a serious, life-threatening disease. Older BMT patients are more likely to develop GVHD than younger patients. The incidence and severity of GVHD is also higher among patients whose bone marrow donor is unrelated or not perfectly matched.

The symptoms of GVHD are many and varied, and the list may at first be overwhelming. Keep in mind however that most patients undergoing an allogeneic BMT with a related HLA-matched donor develop only a mild or moderate case of GVHD, or no GVHD at all. Although GVHD can be life-threatening or fatal, most patients survive the disease without long-term disabling side effects

T-CELLS

T-cells are special white blood cells that recognize foreign matter in the body. T-cells orchestrate attacks on bacteria, viruses and other substances foreign to the body. They can also distinguish "self" from "non-self"—human cells that belong in one person's body and those that do not.

On the surface of many human cells is an inherited set of genetic markers called "human leukocyte antigens" (HLA). Like a fingerprint, no two persons' set of HLA markers are exactly alike (except for identical twins). The T-cells use these HLA markers to distinguish "self" from "non-self." If a "non-self" human cell is encountered in the body, the T-cells quickly activate the immune system to destroy it. The greater the disparity between the body's HLA markers or "tissue type" and that of the foreign human cell, the swifter and more vigorous the attack. (See Chapter 4 for more on the HLA system).

The ability of the immune system's T-cells to distinguish "self" from "non-self" can create a serious problem after allogeneic BMTs. Unless the donor is an identical twin, his or her tissue type (those HLA markers or genetic fingerprints) will differ from that of the patient. The patient's T-cells may identify the donor's bone marrow as "non-self" and attack the donated bone marrow. This is called graft rejection.

To prevent graft rejection, total body irradiation (TBI) and/or drugs such as cyclophosphamide are used to kill the cancerous cells and to suppress a patient's immune system. The radiation and drugs disrupt the ability of T-cells to recognize the donated bone marrow as "non-self" and to launch an immune system attack. (Immune system suppression is not required in autologous BMTs since the bone marrow transfused into the patient is his or her own.)

GVHD

The donor's marrow also contains T-cells. When transplanted into the patient, the donor's T-cells may look at the HLA markers on the patient's cells, identify the cells as "non-self" and unleash an attack on the patient's tissues and organs. Because the patient's own immune system is suppressed prior to the transplant, it cannot launch a counterattack. This condition is called graft-versus-host disease (GVHD). The "graft" is the donated bone marrow and the "host" is the BMT patient or bone marrow recipient.

ACUTE GVHD

Acute GVHD usually occurs during the first three months following

---

STAGES OF ACUTE GVHD

Stage 1 (mild): a skin rash over less than 25% of the body.

Stage 2 (moderate): a skin rash over a more than 25% of the body accompanied by mild liver or stomach and intestinal disorders.

Stage 3 (severe): redness of the skin, similar to a severe sunburn, and moderate liver, stomach and intestinal problems.

Stage 4 (life-threatening): blistering, peeling skin, and severe liver, stomach, and intestinal problems.

---

an allogeneic BMT. T-cells present in the donor's bone marrow at the time of transplant identify the BMT patient as "non-self" and attack the patient's skin, liver, stomach, and/or intestines.

The earliest sign of acute GVHD is often a skin rash that usually first appears on the patient's hands and feet. The rash may spread to other parts of the body and develop into a general redness similar to a sunburn, with peeling or blistering skin. Cramping, nausea, and watery or bloody diarrhea are signs of GVHD in the stomach or intestines. Jaundice (yellowing of the skin and eyes) indicates that acute GVHD has affected the liver.

Physicians grade the severity of acute GVHD according to the number of organs involved and the degree to which they're affected. Acute GVHD may be mild, moderate, severe or life-threatening (see box).

To minimize the risk of graft rejection and GVHD, allogeneic BMT patients are given drugs to prevent GVHD before and after transplant that suppress the immune system. Use of these drugs, however, increases the risk of infection. Precautions taken to limit the patient's exposure to harmful bacteria, viruses and fungi during this period may include special air-filtering equipment in the patient's room, frequent handwashing by visitors, use of masks, gloves and robes by the patient and/or visitors, and elimination of fresh fruits, flowers and vegetables from the patient's environment which may harbor potentially harmful bacteria.

Patients over the age of 30 are more likely to develop acute GVHD than younger patients. Patients receiving marrow from a female donor who has had two or more viable pregnancies also are more likely to develop acute GVHD.

Prevention & Treatment of Acute GVHD

Although GVHD is not yet preventable, steps can be taken to reduce the incidence and severity of GVHD.

Administration of immunosuppressive drugs such as cyclosporine (alone or in combination with steroids) and methotrexate prior to the transplant have proven effective in reducing the incidence and severity of GVHD. They may be administered for several months post-transplant, particularly if acute GVHD progresses to Stage II, or if the patient develops chronic GVHD.

Cyclosporine, steroids and methotrexate weaken the ability of the donor's T-cells to launch an attack against the patient's organs and tissues. These drugs, however, have potential side effects. Cyclosporine can be very toxic to the kidneys, cause increased hair growth on the body, especially facial hair on women, and on rare occasions can result in neurological problems such as seizures, confusion, anxiety, and changes in thought processes. Methotrexate may cause inflammation of the mouth, nose and/or throat. Side effects of steroids include weight gain, fluid retention, elevated blood sugar level, mood swings and/or confused thinking. These side effects are temporary and disappear once use of these drugs is discontinued.

T-cell Depletion

Another technique sometimes used to reduce the severity and incidence of acute GVHD is called "T-cell depletion." Since T-cells identify foreign antigens, researchers hypothesized that removing T-cells from the donor's marrow would decrease the incidence and severity of GVHD. And so it did, reducing the incidence of acute GVHD in leukemic patients from approximately 50 percent to less than 15 percent.

Unfortunately, donor T-cells also appear to play a role in the successful engraftment of the bone marrow in the patient. Thus, while T-cell depletion has decreased the incidence of GVHD in leukemic patients dramatically, the incidence of graft-rejection has risen from near zero in patients whose marrow is not T-cell depleted to 10-30 percent in patients receiving T-cell depleted marrow, resulting in no improvement in long-term survival rates.

In addition, a mild or moderate case of chronic GVHD seems to confer an anti-leukemic effect on the patient. Thus, a little bit of GVHD in leukemic patients may actually be desirable. Completely depleting donor bone marrow of T-cells has not only reduced the incidence of GVHD, but has resulted in relapse rates as high as 65 percent among certain subsets of leukemic patients studied.

BMT centers have tackled this dilemma in several ways. At some centers, less than 100 percent of the T-cells are depleted from the donor's bone marrow prior to infusion. This techniques appears to reduce the incidence of graft-rejection normally associated with complete T-cell depletion, and preserves some of the graft-versus-leukemia effect a mild case of GVHD confers.

Another T-cell depletion technique now under study looks promising. In a trial involving 45 CML (chronic myelogenous leukemia) patients transplanted with marrow from an HLA-matching sibling, the T-cell called CD-8 was selectively purged from the donor's marrow. Using this technique, the incidence of acute GVHD was reduced to 20 percent (from 50 percent when unpurged bone marrow marrow is used), and the high rate of relapse experienced among leukemic patients who receive marrow completely purged of all T-cells did not occur. Graft-rejection was 10 percent, as compared to 10-30 percent when all T-cells are depleted from bone marrow.

CHRONIC GVHD

Chronic GVHD usually develops after the third month post-transplant. Scientists believe that new T-cells produced after the donor's bone marrow has engrafted in the patient may cause chronic GVHD.

Most patients with chronic GVHD experience skin problems that may include a dry itching rash, a change in skin color, and tautness or tightening of the skin. Partial hair loss or premature graying may also occur.

Liver abnormalities are seen in many patients with chronic GVHD. This is usually evidenced by jaundice and abnormal liver test results.

Chronic GVHD can also attack glands in the body that secrete mucous, saliva or other lubricants. Patients with chronic GVHD usually experience dryness or stinging in their eyes because the glands that secrete tears are impaired.

Glands that secrete saliva in the mouth are often affected by chronic GVHD and, less often, those that lubricate the esophagus, making swallowing and eating difficult. It's common for patients with chronic GVHD to experience a burning sensation in their mouths when using toothpaste or eating acidic foods. Good oral hygiene is imperative to minimize the risk of infection.

Chronic GVHD may attack glands that lubricate the stomach lining and intestines, interfering with the body's ability to properly absorb nutrients. Symptoms include heartburn, stomach pain and/or weight loss.

Occasionally patients with chronic GVHD experience "contractures," a tightening of the tendons in joints that makes extending or contracting their arms and legs difficult. Chronic GVHD can also affect the lungs, causing wheezing, bronchitis, or pneumonia.

As is the case with acute GVHD, older patients are more likely to develop chronic GVHD than younger patients. Seventy to 80 percent of patients who develop chronic GVHD will previously have had acute GVHD. Chronic GVHD is also more common in patients whose donor is unrelated or whose marrow is not perfectly matched.

Treatment of Chronic GVHD

Chronic GVHD is usually treatable with steroids such as prednisone, ozothioprine and cyclosporine, which suppress the patient's immune system. Antibiotics such as Bactrim or penicillin or both are usually taken to reduce the risk of infection while chronic GVHD is being treated. In addition, patients may be required to wear face masks while around other people, stay out of crowds, and avoid fresh plants, fruits and vegetables. Patients with chronic GVHD are usually advised to avoid vaccinations with live viruses such as German measles, tetanus, polio, etc. until the GVHD problem is completely resolved and use of immunosuppressive drugs ends.

Researchers have been studying the effectiveness of using other drugs to control chronic GVHD in patients resistant to standard therapy. A recent study found thalidomide to be effective in controlling

---

SYMPTOMS/SIDE EFFECTS OF CHRONIC GVHD

MOST COMMON	LESS COMMON
rash, itching, general redness of skin	skin scarring
dark spots, tautness of skin	partial hair loss, premature graying
jaundice (yellowing of skin & eyes)	severe liver disease
abnormal liver tests	vision impairment
dry, burning eyes	heartburn, stomach pain
dryness or sores in mouth	difficulty swallowing
burning sensation when eating acidic foods	weight loss
bacterial infections	contractures
	difficulty breathing
	bronchitis, pneumonia

chronic GVHD in "high risk" patients (i.e., those likely to develop life-threatening GVHD) with minimal side effects (drowsiness).

LONG TERM CONCERNS

Although most patients recover from GVHD, some symptoms may persist even after the disease has been completely resolved. Patients who've had GVHD usually experience long-term skin sensitivity and must avoid prolonged exposure to sunlight, using strong sunblockers on any exposed skin. Scarring of the skin may also occur.

Eye irritation sometimes persists long-term, and is usually managed with eye drops. Chronic diarrhea and failure of the stomach to properly absorb nutrients may also continue after all clinical signs of GVHD disappear. Some patients experience persistent liver problems and, less frequently, lung problems or contractures.

While GVHD can be a very unpleasant and sometimes fatal complication of an allogeneic BMT, most patients survive the experience without disabling long-term side effects. Scientists are continuing to investigate new ways to prevent and better manage GVHD in the future.

COPING WITH THE STRESS OF GVHD

Since many patients undergoing an allogeneic BMT experience some degree of GVHD, physicians typically discuss GVHD with patients in detail prior to their transplant. Many patients find this discussion overwhelming and frightening, particularly if the risks of GVHD are not put into some perspective. Patients often do not understand that a case of GVHD can be mild, moderate or severe, and that death, disfigurement or permanent disability is not the usual outcome.

A diagnosis of GVHD will affect most patients' emotional and psychological health. Weary of the many complications associated with a BMT, patients often view GVHD as yet another setback that will delay their recovery, and become angry or depressed.

The side effects of drugs used to treat GVHD can further stress a patient's already delicate emotional state. Depression, confusion, anxiety, roller coaster-like mood swings, and exaggerated feelings (anger, excitement, sadness, etc.) disproportionate to the situation are common and can make the GVHD recovery period extremely trying for patients and their loved ones. Keeping in mind that these side effects are temporary can help everyone involved—patient, family and friends—better cope with this period of treatment. In rare instances, medications may be prescribed to stabilize mood swings and reduce anxiety.

Many patients find that building a support system during the recovery period enables them to better cope with the stress of GVHD and other post-transplant complications. This can be done in several ways.

Some patients expand the network of friends and relatives upon whom they rely for help. This can benefit not only the patient, but can give respite to the primary caregivers as well. Family and friends are often eager to help but don't know what to do. Many would be happy to be included on the list of people the patient can call when an understanding, listening ear is needed.

Other patients find support groups organized through their hospital, the American Cancer Society, or similar organizations helpful. Talking with someone who has been through the same experience can lend a unique type of support to patients during this difficult period. Some hospitals and religious organizations also make available one-on-one support services for patients recovering from serious illness. Transplant physicians can usually recommend a social worker who can link patients with various support groups and services.

Often patients find that a professional therapist is very helpful. A therapist can provide a safe environment for the patient to express his or her anger and frustrations, and may have creative suggestions to help a patient cope with his or her stress. Transplant physicians can usually refer patients to therapists experienced in dealing with the complications of BMTs.

Most patients undergoing GVHD treatment experience temporary changes in appearance as a result of the disease or medications used to treat GVHD. Excessive weight gain, a bloated or "moon" face, jaundice (yellow eyes and skin), excessive hair growth on the body, particularly the face and back, and skin irritation which may have the appearance of a mild to severe sunburn can all diminish a patient's self-esteem.

Patients cope with changes in appearance in different ways. Some find it helpful to keep pictures of themselves taken before their illness on hand as a reminder that the physical changes are temporary. Others prefer to avoid reminders of their changed physical appearance altogether.

Because the immune system is suppressed during GVHD recovery, a patient's ability to socialize and interact with the public is limited. Face masks may be required when venturing out of the home and special care must be taken to avoid crowds, people who are ill or those who've been exposed to illness.

Patients do not, however, need to feel like a prisoner in their own home. Seeing movies during daytime hours when attendance is low, shopping in stores during off-hours, eating in restaurants at 5 p.m.

instead of the more crowded 7-8 p.m. dinner hour, etc. allow patients to continue to enjoy public activities during their recovery period without unduly increasing their risk of infection.

Battling GVHD can be a difficult and frustrating experience. For most patients, however, the battle will be temporary and successful.

S usan Mitchell, a BMT patient with aplastic anemia, sums up her experience with GVHD this way: "Sometimes, as I fought off repeated infections and looked at myself in the mirror I thought there would be no end to my misery. But today I'm realizing a happy ending to all of this. Every day is a little brighter and better. My GVHD is gone, my liver is returning to normal, my skin color is back, and I don't itch anymore. I don't do 10K runs yet, but walking seems to suit me well for the time being.

I haven't returned to work yet, but I find my volunteer work at the local hospital and the Heart of America (a bone marrow registry) very rewarding. I take life one day at a time and thank God for giving me loving and supportive family and friends. I never gave up on life and kept a positive attitude. I hope anyone who's facing a BMT finds the same strength I did and never gives up."

CHAPTER 10

Liver Complications

The liver is a complex organ that performs many essential functions not duplicated by other organs. It removes toxins from the bloodstream, manufactures proteins that control blood clotting, stores energy, breaks down drugs, produces a fluid called bile that helps digestion, and rids the body of bilirubin—a pigment produced during the breakup of old red blood cells.

Blood enters the liver through the "portal vein" and the "hepatic artery." It then passes through channels called "sinusoids" that allow contact with liver cells (hepatocytes) that remove and break down drugs, toxins and other waste materials. The cleansed blood flows out of the liver through a network of veins back to the heart.

Hepatocytes also initiate the production of bile, a fluid that contains chemicals needed by the intestines to break down food as well as waste products. It flows through the liver in the opposite direction from blood and enters the gallbladder via bile ducts where it is stored until needed by the small intestine.

If the blood vessels that transport blood through the liver become obstructed or if hepatocytes are damaged, the liver cannot properly rid the body of toxins, drugs, and other waste products. Similarly, if the bile duct becomes obstructed, excess levels of bilirubin, cholesterol and other chemicals will build up in the body, interfering with the function of the liver and other organs.

Liver disorders fall into three categories: (1) those that affect the liver cells (2) those that affect the vessels that transport blood through the liver and (3) those affecting the bile ducts that carry bile from the liver to the gallbladder and intestines. A BMT patient may experience more than one liver disorder at the same time. While some are serious and sometimes fatal, the majority result in only mild or moderate liver damage that is temporary and completely reversible.

The existence of liver disorders pre-transplant can increase the risk of developing severe liver disorders post-transplant. Patients are therefore tested before their BMT for evidence of fungal liver infections, hepatitis

---

SIGNS OF LIVER PROBLEMS

Jaundice (yellowing of skin and eyes)

Tender or swollen liver

Rapid weight gain

Swelling in arms or legs

Fluid accumulation in abdominal cavity

High levels of bilirubin in the blood

High levels of liver enzymes in the blood (SGOT, SGPT and alkaline phosphatase)

Confusion

(inflammation of the liver usually caused by a virus), and gallstones or other obstructions of the bile duct that may need to be removed before the transplant proceeds. These tests also equip physicians with information that may help prevent serious liver problems from developing post-BMT.

A variety of tests are used before, during and after the transplant to determine whether a liver disease is present and whether the disease affects the liver cells, blood vessels, or bile ducts. These tests include a physical examination of the patient to determine the size of the liver, blood tests that measure the level in the bloodstream of bilirubin and proteins produced by the liver, "imaging tests" such as ultrasound and CT X-rays ("CAT scans") that provide a picture of the liver, its blood vessels and bile ducts, and liver biopsy.

While in the hospital, daily measurements of a patient's abdominal girth, weight, and blood levels of bilirubin and other liver enzymes aid in the early detection of liver problems. Daily examination of the patient for signs of jaundice or swelling also helps the medical staff detect liver problems.

DURING THE FIRST THREE MONTHS AFTER A BMT

Veno-Occlusive Disease (VOD)

Veno-occlusive disease is a potentially serious liver problem caused by the high dose of chemotherapy and/or radiation given to patients before the transplant. In patients with VOD, the blood vessels that carry blood through the liver become swollen and obstructed. This impairs the liver's ability to remove toxins, drugs and other waste products from the bloodstream. Pressure and fluids build up in the liver, causing swelling and tenderness of the liver. The kidneys may retain excess water and salt, causing fluid to build up in the body and swelling of the legs, arms and abdomen to occur.

In severe cases of VOD, build up of fluid that has leaked into the abdominal cavity may also put pressure on the lungs and impair breathing. Toxins that are not processed out of the blood by the liver may affect how the brain functions and confusion may result (although confusion is a symptom of other, less serious post-BMT problems as well). The kidneys, heart and lungs may also fail.

Symptoms of VOD are usually first seen one to four weeks after the start of the "conditioning" or "preparative" regimen—the chemotherapy and/or radiation administered to patients immediately before the transplant. VOD can be difficult to diagnose, however, since its symptoms are signs of other liver disorders as well. The symptoms include jaundice, an enlarged liver, pain or tenderness in the area of the liver (located on the right side of the body under the lower rib cage), rapid weight gain, swelling (edema), and accumulation of fluid in the abdominal cavity (ascites). If an enlarged liver AND sudden weight gain AND jaundice occur early after transplant and cannot be explained by other causes, VOD probably exists.

There currently is no proven preventive therapy for VOD. When VOD is diagnosed, the medical team will take steps to prevent the more serious complications from developing. These include minimizing or eliminating the use of certain drugs that can worsen the problem, relieving the buildup of fluids in tissues and organs with diuretics or dialysis, restricting the intake of salt, carefully monitoring the volume of fluids in the body, and transfusing the patient with packed red blood cells to keep the circulating blood volume high until VOD has run its course.

Patients with malignant diseases such as leukemia, lymphomas and solid tumors are more likely to develop severe veno-occlusive disease post-transplant than patients with non-malignant disorders such as aplastic anemia or an immune deficiency disease. This is because the conditioning regimen for these patients usually involves stronger doses of chemotherapy and/or radiation than those administered to patients with non-malignant disorders. While the stronger doses of chemotherapy and/or radiation increase the likelihood that cancerous cells will be destroyed, they are also much more toxic to the liver.

Other factors that increase the risk of developing severe VOD include pre-transplant hepatitis, the presence of a fever resulting from an infection anywhere in the body immediately before or during the course of the preparative regimen, and use of mis-matched or unrelated donor marrow. Patients undergoing a second transplant also may be at higher risk of developing VOD than others.

In most cases, VOD is mild or moderate, and the liver damage is completely reversible. Severe VOD, however, is usually fatal.

Acute GVHD of the Liver

Patients undergoing allogeneic BMTs are at risk of developing liver damage from acute graft-versus-host disease.

In GVHD, the bone marrow provided by a donor (the graft) attacks the tissues and organs of the BMT patient (the host). Acute GVHD occurs during the first three months post-transplant. Chronic GVHD, a separate disease, occurs after the third month post-transplant.

Acute GVHD of the liver affects small bile ducts, interfering with the flow of bile out of the liver. Bile duct damage may be mild, moderate or severe. Doctors measure the level of bilirubin and an enzyme called alkaline phosphatase in the bloodstream to determine the severity of the disease.

The signs of acute GVHD of the liver include jaundice, mild liver tenderness, and increased levels of bilirubin and alkaline phosphatase in the bloodstream.

To prevent the development of acute GVHD, patients undergoing an allogeneic BMT are usually given drugs such as methotrexate, cyclosporine and occasionally prednisone. Some centers use a procedure called "T-cell depletion" to remove certain types of lymphocytes (white blood cells) from donor marrow before the BMT to prevent acute GVHD. If acute GVHD occurs, cyclosporine and increased dosages of prednisone are the usual treatment.

Use of unrelated donor marrow increases the risk of developing acute GVHD of the liver. Patients transplanted with donor marrow that is not a perfect (6-antigen) match are also at increased risk of developing acute GVHD of the liver.

Bloodstream Infections

Abnormalities in bile flow are sometimes triggered by infections in the bloodstream. This condition (sometimes called cholangitis lenta) is not an infection of the liver itself, but the liver's response to an infection elsewhere in the body. Symptoms include jaundice, an increased level of bilirubin and sometimes alkaline phosphatase in the blood.

The bile flow abnormalities resulting from cholangitis lenta can usually be reversed by treating the underlying bloodstream infection with antibiotics.

Fungal Liver Disease

Fungal liver disease is a serious post-transplant complication. The

Candida species of fungus, which resides in the intestines, is the usual cause of fungal liver disease. Normally, the spread of this fungus is kept in check by beneficial bacteria that reside in the body and by the immune system.

In the first few weeks post-transplant, antibiotics given to BMT patients to destroy harmful bacteria also destroy the beneficial bacteria that keep the spread of Candida fungi in check. The fungi may multiply and get into the bloodstream. If the patient's immune system isn't strong enough to destroy them, the fungi may set up housekeeping in the liver, spleen or kidneys.

Symptoms of fungal liver infection include persistent fever, a tender swollen liver, and an elevated level of alkaline phosphatase in the blood.

Patients with fungal infections in their intestine or bloodstream after transplant are at greatest risk of developing fungal liver disease. Patients who have persistent low granulocyte (a type of white blood cell) counts and those receiving prednisone therapy for graft-versus-host disease are also more likely to develop fungal liver infections than others.

Fungal infections are very difficult to treat, particularly when the immune system is weak. Amphotericin B and fluconazole are two drugs that have shown some effectiveness in treating fungal liver infection.

Drug-induced Liver Injury

Several drugs administered to BMT patients to treat infections, GVHD, nausea, and high blood pressure as well as some sedatives and pain medications can cause or aggravate liver injury. While a frequent cause of mild liver injury, these drugs seldom cause severe liver damage. The signs of drug injury are jaundice and abnormal levels of bilirubin and liver enzymes (SGOT, SGPT and alkaline phosphatase) in the blood.

Prolonged periods of intravenous feeding (also called hyperalimentation or total parenteral nutrition [TPN]) can also cause mild liver problems in BMT patients. These problems are temporary and include liver inflammation, abnormal bile flow and fat accumulation in the liver. The problems are usually corrected by reducing the patient's intravenous caloric intake and returning the patient to oral feeding. If oral feeding is not possible, varying the content of the intravenous feeding may help.

Viral Hepatitis

Occasionally, viral hepatitis (inflammation of the liver caused by a virus) occurs in BMT patients during the first three months post-transplant. It is usually caused by the hepatitis B or C virus but can also be caused by other viruses such as Adenovirus, Herpes simplex virus, Varicella zoster virus, Echovirus, Cytomegalovirus (CMV), and Epstein-Barr virus.

Liver inflammation caused by the hepatitis B or C virus is usually mild and seldom results in death. The hepatitis B or C virus is often in a patient's bloodstream as a result of multiple blood transfusions received during earlier treatment. BMT centers now screen blood products given to BMT patients for CMV and the hepatitis A, B and C viruses.

Liver infections caused by other viruses (Adenovirus, Herpes simplex virus, Varicella zoster virus) rarely cause severe liver damage and death. Early diagnosis of these infections is important since therapies available to treat these viruses are most effective during the early stages of infection. (See Chapter 8 for more on viral infections.)

Biliary Disease

When patients stop eating for an extended period of time (e.g. when they are fed intravenously) the gallbladder, which stores bile and squeezes it into the intestine after meals, does not empty. The bile becomes thick and granular, creating "biliary sludge." The sludge can obstruct the bile duct and interfere with the flow of bile to the small intestine.

Symptoms of this problem include pain after eating, inflammation of the gallbladder, fever, and gallstones. The problem usually resolves itself once the patient begins eating normally. In rare cases, an infection of the bile duct or inflammation of the pancreas may result.

AFTER THE THIRD MONTH POST-TRANSPLANT

Liver problems are much less common after the third month post-transplant than during the first three months. Patients who have had acute GVHD or viral hepatitis B or C during the first three months post-transplant are more likely to experience liver disorders after the third month post-transplant than others. Most liver disorders occurring during this period are mild or moderate and are not fatal.

Chronic GVHD of the Liver

Like acute GVHD, chronic GVHD can attack the small bile ducts and interfere with the flow of bile from the liver to the intestines. Symptoms include jaundice and elevated levels of alkaline phosphatase and bilirubin in the blood. Chronic GVHD of the liver is a potential complication of allogeneic transplants. It is not a complication of autologous (self) or syngeneic (identical twin) BMTs.

Chronic GVHD usually results in only mild or moderate liver damage, which can cause a mild loss of appetite. Most cases can be successfully treated with immunosuppressive drugs such as prednisone and cyclosporine. Severe cases may be treated with higher dosages of these drugs as well as Actigall (ursodeoxycholic acid) or Imuran (azathioprine). Patients who have had acute GVHD of the liver are at greater risk for developing chronic GVHD of the liver than other allogeneic BMT patients.

Chronic Viral Hepatitis

Viruses can linger in the body long after symptoms of acute infection disappear and infections can recur long after the first episode. This is particularly true if the body's immune system is not functioning normally as is often the case with BMT patients, particularly those with chronic GVHD.

Viral hepatitis (usually caused by the hepatitis C virus) can flare up many months post-transplant. Chronic viral hepatitis is often difficult to treat. Some chronic liver infections caused by the hepatitis C virus can be successfully treated with the drug interferon. This drug, however, must be used with great caution, especially in patients with chronic GVHD. Interferon can suppress the patient's white blood cell count and increase the risk of bloodstream infections.

Fungal Liver Disease

On rare occasions, fungal liver disease similar to that seen in patients during the first three months post-transplant develops after the third month post-transplant. It is most often seen in patients whose bone marrow contains low levels of granulocytes and in patients with chronic GVHD. Symptoms and treatment of these fungal infections are the same as those associated with fungal infections that occur during first three months post-transplant.

CHAPTER 11

Infertility

One of the more disturbing pieces of information BMT patients may hear prior to their transplant is that their ability to achieve a pregnancy post-BMT will be impaired. For persons who have not yet begun or wish to expand their family, this news can be devastating.

It's not the BMT itself but the high-dose chemotherapy and/or radiation administered prior to the BMT that often damages reproductive cells. Most chemotherapy agents and radiation are incapable of distinguishing between normal and diseased cells and may damage delicate reproductive cells while eradicating the disease.

Not all patients undergoing a BMT experience infertility. The likelihood of infertility varies according to the patient's age, gender, sexual maturity, the type and amount of chemotherapy and/or radiation administered, and preventive steps taken during treatment. Thus, many patients with leukemia or Hodgkin's disease often are infertile before a BMT, as a result of prior chemotherapy.

Since post-transplant infertility is not a life-threatening condition, little medical attention has focused on the problem to date. As the survival rates for BMT patients continue to improve, however, "quality of life" issues like fertility are becoming a major concern for BMT survivors.

Fortunately, there are options available to couples who wish to have children post-transplant. Besides adoption, medically assisted reproduction techniques such as sperm-banking, cryogenic preservation (freezing) of embryos, artificial insemination, in-vitro fertilization, and sperm and embryo donation provide hope for patients who are infertile following their BMT. Religious, ethical, medical and financial concerns may temper the range of options an individual is willing to consider. However, understanding the options in advance of your BMT treatment will enable you to better plan for children post-transplant, and relieve some of the stress associated with the prospect of infertility.

STEPS TO PREGNANCY

Achieving a pregnancy is a delicately timed, intricate process. Normally, both partners must have functioning reproductive organs that enable the woman to produce a mature egg that can be fertilized by healthy male sperm. The fertilized egg must then migrate to the woman's uterus and implant in the lining (endometrium) where it will begin to mature into a fetus.

Eggs are produced in the ovaries. At the beginning of each menstrual cycle, follicle stimulating hormone (FSH) is released by the pituitary gland located near the brain. FSH causes immature eggs (oocytes) contained in fluid filled sacs (follicles) inside the ovaries to begin to mature—one egg per follicle. Although 100-150 oocytes may begin to mature each cycle, only one egg in one ovary will usually reach full maturity around the 12th to 14th day of the cycle.

The developing eggs release a hormone into the bloodstream called estrogen. Estrogen, among other things, causes the lining of the uterus to thicken in preparation to receive an embryo. The estrogen level will peak when the single egg destined to mature that cycle is fully developed, stimulating the pituitary gland to produce "luteinizing hor-

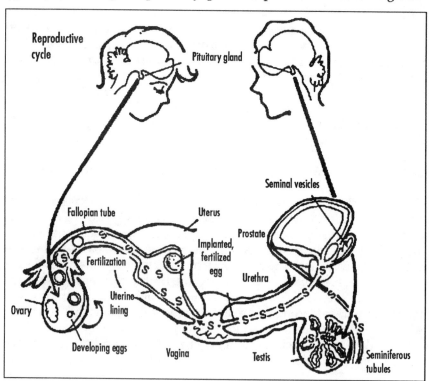

mone" (LH). LH triggers the release of the mature egg into the fallopian tube. The enveloping outer layer of the follicle (after ovulation, called the corpus luteum) remains in the ovary and produces progesterone. Progesterone and other hormones secreted by the corpus luteum fortify the uterine lining so that it can receive and nurture the embryo.

The fallopian tubes connect the ovaries to the uterus. At the junction of the ovaries and fallopian tubes are small fingerlike "fimbria" that pick up the mature egg and move it into the fallopian tube where fertilization occurs. Since the egg must be fertilized within 24 hours of entering the fallopian tube, there is a very small "window of opportunity" for sperm to enter the woman's uterus via the vagina, migrate to the fallopian tube, and fuse with the egg to create an embryo. Although as many as 400 million sperm may be ejaculated during sexual intercourse, only a few hundred will successfully reach the fallopian tubes.

Once the sperm fertilizes the egg, the resulting single cell embryo begins to divide and multiply. By the 4th or 5th day, when it enters the uterus, it's composed of more than 100 cells. The embryo must implant in the uterine lining in order to continue growing. This usually occurs five to seven days after fertilization and is the beginning of a pregnancy. If implantation occurs, the embryo will discharge a hormone called "human chorionic gonadotropin" (HCG) that signals the ovaries to continue producing estrogen and progesterone to support the uterine lining. (Early pregnancy tests measure the level of HCG in the blood.) If the embryo fails to implant, it degenerates and is destroyed by the immune system.

SPERM PRODUCTION

Sperm are manufactured in microscopic threadlike tubes in the testicles called "seminiferous tubules." The same hormones that stimulate the production of eggs in women's ovaries—FSH and LH—stimulate production of sperm in men.

The cells on the inside walls of the seminiferous tubules generate millions of new immature sperm cells (spermatocytes) daily. A spermatocyte divides twice as it migrates to the center of the seminiferous tubule, where the resulting four "spermatids" mature into tadpole shaped sperm. The heads of the sperm contain the genetic information that will fuse with the woman's egg, as well as chemicals that enable the sperm to penetrate the outer shell of the egg.

The sperm leave the testicles and move through a long coiled tube called the "epididymis" where they mature and are stored. Upon ejaculation, the sperm move to pouches behind the bladder called "seminal vesicles" where fluid from the seminal vesicles and the prostate gland is added to create semen (98 percent fluid, 2 percent sperm). The fluid provides nutrients to sustain and protect the sperm. The semen then passes through the "urethra"—a tube in the penis connecting both the bladder and the seminal vesicles to outside the body.

During sexual intercourse, sperm are ejaculated into a woman's vagina near the "cervix" or the entrance to the uterus. The sperm must navigate through the cervix and uterus into the fallopian tubes where fertilization of an egg can occur. Upon meeting the egg, one sperm will use the chemicals stored in its head to penetrate the shell of the egg and drill to the center where its genetic material (DNA) will fuse with that of the egg, creating an embryo.

CHEMOTHERAPY & RADIATION

Chemotherapy, especially combination chemotherapy, can damage or destroy the cells in testes and ovaries from which sperm and eggs evolve. Radiation causes similar problems, and can damage the uterine lining or fallopian tubes as well.

Infertility caused by chemotherapy and/or radiation may be temporary or permanent, and may occur at low doses as well as the higher doses administered pre-BMT. Patients who have undergone standard chemotherapy and/or radiation treatment for their disease prior to considering a BMT are often already infertile at the time of their BMT.

A class of chemotherapy drugs called "alkylating agents" is especially toxic to reproductive cells. They include cyclophosphamide (Cytoxan), ifosfamide, melphalan (l-Pam), mechlorethamine hydrochloride (nitrogen mustard), thiotepa, and busulfan (Myleran). Other chemotherapy drugs such as carmustine (BCNU), chlorambucil, cytosine arabinoside (cytarabine) (ARA-C), cisplatin (CDDP), doxorubicin (Adriamycin), procarbazine, and vinblastine (Velban) can also cause infertility.

In general, younger patients are less likely than older patients to develop permanent infertility as a result of standard chemotherapy treatment. This is particularly true of pre-pubertal patients and women. Infertility is often related to the type and dosage of chemotherapy administered, with higher cumulative dosages being more toxic to reproductive cells than lower dosages.

Patients with early-stage Hodgkin's disease can sometimes be treated with ABVD (Adriamycin, bleomycin, vinblastine, and DTIC or dacarbazine), which is equally efficacious, but less toxic to reproductive cells than another chemotherapy regimen used to treat the disease called

DRUGS THAT CAN CAUSE INFERTILITY

Drugs	Diseases they are used to treat
Cytoxan:	leukemias, aplastic anemia, lymphomas, breast and ovarian cancer
Ifosfamide:	sarcomas, breast and urologic cancers
L-Pam:	multiple myeloma
Nitrogen Mustard:	Hodgkin's disease
Thiotepa:	breast cancer
Busulfan:	leukemias
BCNU:	brain tumors
Chlorambucil:	leukemias, lymphomas
ARA-C:	leukemias, lymphomas
Cisplatin:	head & neck tumors, lung cancer, breast and ovarian cancer, lymphomas, testicular cancer
Adriamycin:	breast & ovarian cancer, lymphomas, Hodgkin's disease, sarcomas, small cell lung cancer
Procarbazine:	Hodgkin's disease
Velban:	Hodgkin's disease, lymphomas, breast & testicular cancer

MOPP (nitrogen mustard, Oncovin, procarbazine and prednisone). This less toxic therapy is not an option, however, when the disease has progressed to the stage where a BMT is required.

Researchers have theorized that administering hormones in conjunction with chemotherapy to suppress reproductive organ functions during treatment may reduce the incidence of permanent infertility. This theory, however, has yet to be confirmed by large clinical trials.

Most of the information known about the effect of chemotherapy on reproductive cells has been drawn from studies of patients receiving lower doses of chemotherapy than typically administered to BMT patients. In the one study conducted on BMT patients (with aplastic anemia) who received high-dose chemotherapy pre-transplant (200 mg/kg of cyclophosphamide without total body irradiation), all females under the age of 26 regained fertility post-transplant, while only one-third of females over the age of 25, and two-thirds of all males regained fertility post-BMT. (These results should not be extrapolated to patients undergoing different high-dose chemotherapy regimens pre-BMT for different diseases.)

Use of radiation in combination with chemotherapy increases the risk of infertility, even in younger patients. Patient age, sex, stage of sexual maturity and total cumulative dosage affect the likelihood of infertility after radiation therapy. Few patients who receive total body irradiation pre-BMT remain fertile post-transplant.

Although data on pregnancies post-BMT are not systematically gathered and centrally reported, at least 64 pregnancies by BMT patients are known to have occurred.

MEDICALLY ASSISTED REPRODUCTION

Couples who wish to bear children post-transplant may benefit by recent advances in medically assisted reproduction technology. While not always successful, assisted reproduction provides men with the opportunity to contribute to the genetic make-up of their child and allows women to be the biological (and sometimes genetic) mother of the child.

Artificial Insemination

For men undergoing chemotherapy and a BMT, sperm-banking is the best way to preserve their ability to be a biological father in the future. Artificial insemination is a procedure in which male sperm are injected into a woman's vagina at the point in her monthly cycle when the mature egg is most likely to have been released into the fallopian tube. Since it can be difficult to precisely predict when the egg will reach the fallopian tube, artificial insemination is often repeated over two consecutive days to maximize the likelihood of success. If the sperm fertilizes the egg, and the resulting embryo migrates to the uterus and implants in the lining, a pregnancy begins.

Frozen sperm have been successfully used in artificial insemination. Thus, men facing the possibility of infertility post-transplant may wish to "bank" some of their sperm prior to the BMT to enable fertilization of their partner's egg at some later date.

Sperm banking is a relatively simple procedure. Typically, several ejaculates of sperm are collected over a one to three week period and frozen or "cryopreserved" in sterile containers. On average, six vials of sperm are obtained per ejaculate. (One or two vials are needed for each artificial insemination cycle.) Although the sperm count and motility (ability of sperm to propel themselves forward) of ejaculates from pre-BMT patients are sometimes lower than values typically required by a sperm bank for cryopreservation, they nonetheless can usually be frozen and later used successfully in artificial insemination cycles.

Charges for sperm banking include a fee to process the semen sample ($100-$500 per ejaculate), an annual storage fee ($150-$400 per patient), and packing and shipping charges. Charges for the artificial insemination procedure itself include a fee to thaw and prepare the sperm ($100-$200 per vial) and the physician's fee. Health insurance plans may cover all, some or none of these charges.

Donor Sperm

If a patient's sperm is not frozen prior to the BMT, it is still possible to achieve a pregnancy via artificial insemination using donor sperm. The sperm may be provided by a donor known to the couple, or obtained anonymously from a sperm bank.

Some sperm banks that supply anonymous donor sperm samples will provide non-identifying information about the donor e.g. age, race, hair and eye color, religion, occupation, hobbies, etc. It's recommended that anonymous donor sperm be frozen for at least six months prior to use so that comprehensive testing for HIV (the AIDS virus) can be conducted. The cost of donor sperm varies from $25 to $125 per vial, depending on the sperm bank.

Success Rate

According to a 1988 study prepared by the U.S. Office of Technology Assessment, 65,000 infants are born annually through artificial insemination. Individual clinics report that 50 to 90 percent of women who undergo artificial insemination for a 12-month period using fresh sperm, or an 18-month period using frozen sperm, become pregnant.

A successful artificial insemination program requires a physician who's skilled in determining when a woman will ovulate so that the timing of the insemination maximizes the likelihood that the sperm will fertilize the ovum. Handling frozen sperm requires more physician and laboratory skill than working with fresh sperm since techniques and temperatures used in thawing, cleaning and incubating the sperm sample affect the number of sperm that survive the thawing process. Fifty to 75 percent of sperm in a cryopreserved sample typically survive the thawing.

In addition to a viable sperm sample, artificial insemination requires normal reproductive functions on the part of the woman to be inseminated. If she has difficulty producing a healthy egg, if her uterus is not properly prepared during the reproductive cycle to receive and nurture the embryo, if there is scarring in her fallopian tubes or if she is over the age of 39, successful artificial insemination may not be possible without further medical intervention.

In-Vitro Fertilization

Although it's possible to freeze male sperm, it's very difficult to successfully freeze unfertilized eggs. No live births have yet been reported using eggs that were frozen prior to fertilization. An option analogous to sperm-banking, therefore, is not now available to women facing post-BMT infertility. It is, however, possible for women with post-BMT ovarian failure to attempt in-vitro fertilization (IVF) with donor eggs.

In IVF several mature eggs provided by a woman are combined in a laboratory dish with male sperm, where fertilization occurs. The resulting embryos are then transferred to the woman's uterus. If an embryo implants in the uterine lining a pregnancy begins.

Initially IVF was used to help women whose ovaries were functional (were capable of producing eggs) but who nonetheless had difficulty conceiving a child. More recently, women with ovarian failure, women of advanced age, and women who have concerns about the integrity of their eggs following chemotherapy or radiation treatment have used IVF with donor eggs to achieve pregnancy. Although IVF with donor eggs does not enable a woman to contribute to the genetic make-up of the child, she does provide the nurturing womb during the nine months of pregnancy required for successful childbirth, and is the biological (as distinguished from genetic) mother of the child.

Donors in IVF programs may either be someone known to the couple or anonymous. Some IVF donor programs require couples to provide their own egg donors, others strictly use anonymous donors, and still others will work with either.

To secure the necessary eggs, the donor is injected with drugs such as human menopausal gonadatropin (Pergonal), FSH (Metrodin), HCG, or leuprolide (Lupron) over a 10 to 21 day period to stimulate several eggs to mature in the ovaries. The patient into whose uterus the fertilized eggs will be transferred is put on a daily regimen of oral estrogen and progesterone injections to prepare the uterus to receive and nurture the embryos.

When the donor's eggs have matured, they are "harvested" through a minor surgical procedure called ultrasound guided needle aspiration, or through another surgical procedure requiring general anesthesia called laparoscopy. The eggs are combined with male sperm in a laboratory dish and incubated for 18-24 hours. The resulting embryos are transferred to the recipient's uterus using a thin catheter with a syringe on the end. Typically three to five embryos are transferred during this five to 10 minute non-surgical procedure.

Two variations on IVF are "GIFT" (gamete intrafallopian tube transfer) and "ZIFT" (zygote intrafallopian tube transfer). In GIFT, male sperm and donor eggs are combined after retrieval and immediately injected into the fallopian tubes so that fertilization can occur in its normal environment rather than in the laboratory. In ZIFT, the eggs are fertilized by sperm in the laboratory and then transferred to the fallopian tubes rather than the uterus as in IVF. While some clinics report higher success rates with GIFT and ZIFT than with IVF, many experts argue these results are biased by patient selection, and do not control for the skill of the laboratory personnel who handle the fertilization process during IVF.

Charges for a single IVF, GIFT or ZIFT cycle range from $6,000 to $12,000 depending on the clinic involved, financial arrangements with the donor, and travel/lodging costs. All, some or none of these charges may be covered by your health insurance. Follow-up expenses (e.g. pregnancy tests, prenatal care, etc.) are usually covered by insurance in the same way that standard pregnancies are covered.

Frozen Embryos
Although it is not currently feasible to freeze unfertilized female eggs, it is possible to freeze fertilized eggs or embryos. In most IVF programs, any embryos in excess of those needed for transfer to the uterus that cycle are frozen for later use.

At least one clinic, Center for Reproductive Medicine & Infertility at Cornell Medical College, New York City, has initiated an experimental program that affords women who are about to undergo chemotherapy and/or radiation the opportunity to freeze their own fertilized eggs prior to treatment. Eight women have participated in the program to date. Although fertilized eggs have been successfully frozen, none of the patients has sufficiently recovered from her disease thus far to attempt an IVF transfer with the frozen embryos.

Success Rate of IVF with Donor Eggs
According to figures released by the US IVF Registry, 48 clinics performed IVF with donor eggs on 328 women in 1989. Of the 377 IVF-donor embryo transfer cycles attempted, 21 percent resulted in live births. Success rates for IVF embryo transfer cycles using frozen embryos were lower (8 percent), with 10 of the 110 reporting clinics accounting for 54 percent of all live births.

Several factors influence IVF-donor embryo transfer success rates, and great care should be exercised in interpreting and comparing statistics from individual clinics. In addition to the skill of the physician and laboratory personnel, the age of the woman undergoing IVF, the age and responsiveness of the donor to ovary-stimulating drugs, and male sperm factor problems all influence an IVF success rate.

Choosing a Program

Finding a competent assisted reproduction program that suits your needs requires research, careful analysis, and guidance from an informed gynecologist or infertility specialist. You may need to travel out of state to find a program appropriate for you.

The Society for Assisted Reproductive Technology (SART) sets minimum standards that member programs must follow regarding cryopreservation of sperm and embryos, artificial insemination and in-vitro fertilization. SART also requires member programs to meet certain criteria regarding training and experience of physicians and laboratory personnel working in the program, and to publicly release data on their clinic's success rates. The American Fertility Society (AFS) can provide you with a copy of these standards, a list of SART members, clinic-specific success rates for IVF (data does not include IVF cycles using donor eggs) and can identify those members with IVF-donor egg programs.

When selecting a fertility program, ask how many artificial insemination or IVF-donor egg cycles have been attempted by the clinic, and how many live births have resulted. When evaluating individual programs, it's helpful to focus on their success rate with couples whose specific fertility problems, medical history, and age mirror your own, as well as the program's overall success rate. Be wary of established programs that provide only national success rates or data on other clinics' experiences rather than their own.

If you're considering IVF with donor eggs and are unable to supply your own donor, ask whether the fertility clinic provides donors. If the answer is yes, find out how many active donors are currently available and how long you must wait before being matched. Some programs say they have donors available, but in fact are still trying to locate some. Others have numerous donors on call who can be matched with you in a reasonably short period of time. Ask how donors are recruited, what medical and other evaluations are conducted, and what you can specify about the donor with whom you're to be matched.

Fertility programs also differ in the level of emotional support and psychological counseling they provide. At some clinics, psychologists and social workers are an integral part of the program, while at others no such support services exist. Medically assisted reproduction can be a trying experience and you may find such support services important.

Emotional Considerations

Before deciding to attempt medically assisted reproduction, couples need to consider the BMT patient's prognosis for long-term survival, whether the healthy partner is prepared to handle single-parenting (either temporarily or long-term) if relapse or death occurs, and the impact of a relapse or death on the child. Patients should also discuss with their physician whether pregnancy could exacerbate their medical condition.

As with BMTs, medically assisted reproduction offers no guarantee—just a chance of pregnancy. It may take several tries before pregnancy is achieved and some couples may never be successful. Moreover, if pregnancy is achieved, the usual possibilities of miscarriage and fetal abnormalities exist. Couples should be prepared for disappointment as well as success.

Programs involving donor eggs or sperm can create additional dilemmas. Will the couple be more comfortable with a known donor or an anonymous donor? Should relatives and friends be told if a donor is used? What will the child want to know about the donor who helped make conception possible?

For couples who choose to produce and freeze embryos for future use, the question of what to do with the embryos if one partner dies or if the marriage is dissolved must be addressed. Should the embryos be destroyed? Should they be donated to another infertile couple? Should one partner in a divorce be awarded custody rights? These are emotionally charged legal and ethical questions that couples may find very difficult to address, particularly if the decisions must be made at the same time a BMT or other cancer therapy is being considered.

THE ADOPTION OPTION

Successful adoption requires a major commitment of time, resources, and emotional energy. There are two adoption strategies to consider: agency-assisted adoption and private adoption.

Agency-Assisted Adoption

Several agencies facilitate adoptions in the U.S. They vary greatly in the number of children available for placement, fees, and requirements for adoptive parents.

"Traditional" agencies (e.g., Catholic Charities, Jewish Children's

Bureau, and several non-denominational agencies) are the least costly way to adopt a child, but facilitate the fewest adoptions annually. They have the most restrictive requirements for adoptive parents regarding religion, marital status, marital time, age, employment status, proof of infertility, the number of other children in the home, and health status. "Non-traditional" agencies are more expensive but have more children available for placement and are more flexible in the type of adoptive parent with whom they're willing to work.

Some agencies specialize in out-of-state adoptions, international adoptions, or adoption of "waiting children" e.g., minority or biracial children, older children, children with special physical or emotional needs, and children who are part of a sibling group. Persons willing to adopt "waiting children" can often locate a child more quickly than those with stricter age, ethnic or health requirements.

Most agencies offer adoptive parents the security of knowing that birth mothers have been screened for medical fitness, history of drug/alcohol abuse, etc. and have been counseled in and assisted with prenatal care. Agencies also usually counsel birth mothers regarding their decision to place the child with adoptive parents and discuss with them all other options in an effort to ensure that the mother is making an informed decision.

In most states a preplacement "home study" to license the adoptive parents is required for any agency-assisted, out-of-state, or international adoption. Adoptive parents must provide written proof of medical fitness as part of the home study. Former BMT patients may find it difficult or impossible to satisfy the medical requirements of a home study and may therefore need to pursue "private adoption." However some states require a home study for private adoption as well).

Private Adoption

It's very common and usually much faster for adoptive parents to locate a birth mother on their own rather than rely on agencies. In most states, there are attorneys and/or adoption consultants who specialize in counseling adoptive parents on how to search for birth mothers and how to screen and work with prospective birth mothers during the prenatal period. The consultants also provide guidance on legal issues such as the level of financial assistance (if any) allowed by the state to be paid to the birth mother during the prenatal period, custody rights of the birth mother and father, and the proper procedure for legally finalizing the adoption after birth.

Great care is advised when selecting an attorney to assist with a private adoption. Most states have strict laws against "baby brokering" that limit the level of attorney involvement in finding babies for adoptive parents. Attorneys who seek out birth mothers and pressure them into placing their child in an adoptive home, who make illegal payments to birth mothers to secure children, or who mishandle legal notices and filings required to finalize the adoption process place adoptive parents at risk of losing the child if the birth mother (or father) later seeks reversal of the adoption.

Cost

The cost of adoption can range from as little as $8,000 to $30,000, with most falling in the range of $10,000 to $15,000. Factors influencing the price include whether you use an agency or adopt privately, whether the adoption is in-state, out-of-state or international, the extent to which the birth mother's medical and personal expenses must be (and can legally be) financed by the adoptive parents during the prenatal period, and whether or not your insurance or employee benefit plan covers some adoption-related expenses.

Emotional Considerations

Finding a baby to adopt can be a lengthy and frustrating process. It may take many months to locate a birth mother willing to place her child in your custody. Moreover in many states, birth mothers (and sometimes fathers) can, for a period of time after the child has been placed in an adoptive home, rescind their decision to allow the child to be adopted. These legal challenges can be very traumatic for everyone involved.

"Open" adoptions in which the birth parents and adoptive parents meet and/or learn something about each other are now quite common. Some birth mothers may want ongoing contact with the child after birth as a condition of adoption. Adoptive parents need to assess the level of "openness" (if any) with which they and the adoptive child will be most comfortable.

CHAPTER 12

Insurance and Bone Marrow Transplants

There's a tug-of-war going on between some insurance companies and hospitals with BMT patients caught in the middle. On the one hand, hospitals are striving to provide the most effective, state of the art health care for their patients. On the other hand, insurance companies are fighting to contain escalating health care costs. The patients are simply fighting to stay alive.

Between 1988 and 1991 more than 200 people were unable to undergo a BMT because their insurance company would not cover the cost of the procedure. Many more had their BMT delayed as they attempted to persuade insurers to pay for the BMT or tried to raise the funds on their own. The good news is that the situation is improving. The bad news is that persuading insurers to cover a BMT often involves a long, arduous fight—a fight most BMT patients are unprepared to undertake alone.

A 1991 BMT Newsletter survey of transplant centers found that an autologous BMT—a BMT in which the patient is his/her own bone marrow donor—is the type of BMT most frequently resisted by insurance companies, particularly if it is for treatment of breast cancer or other solid tumors. The survey also found that, despite insurers' initial refusal to pre-approve an autologous BMT, correspondence from the patient's physician that included studies showing the effectiveness of BMTs in treating the patient's disease, second opinions from other medical experts in the field, and evidence that other medical authorities endorse the practice was often successful in reversing the insurer's initial denial of BMT coverage. Intervention by employers and legal action have also been effective in compelling payment.

Insurance reimbursement for BMTs using mis-matched donors (donors whose bone marrow is not a perfect genetic match with the patient's) was also cited by survey respondents as a problem. The costs incurred in locating a suitable bone marrow donor, performing physical exams on the donor, and extracting the donor's bone marrow were frequently cited by respondents as expenses insurance failed to reimburse.

What's the bottom line? Don't assume your insurance company will cover any or all costs associated with your BMT. Knowing your rights, understanding your insurance policy, enlisting the help of your employer and having a physician who's willing to work closely with you to persuade your insurer to cover your BMT is essential. If you're one of the many persons whose insurance company will pay for your BMT without a fight, be thankful. If not, remember: when your insurance company says "no" don't take no for an answer. Read on for strategies you can use to secure insurance coverage of your BMT.

WHAT TYPES OF INSURANCE ARE AVAILABLE?

There are four kinds of health insurance plans prevalent today: private insurance, self-insured plans, health maintenance organizations (HMOs) and government programs.

Private Insurance

Private insurance is the most common type of plan. In exchange for an annual premium payment, the insurance company reimburses certain health care expenses incurred by the patient. Reimbursable expenses are spelled out in a written plan description which, by law, must be provided to each plan participant. Private insurance may be purchased by an individual, or by an employer or association on behalf of its employees/members.

Persons with private health insurance can choose the doctor or hospital who will provide them with care. Reimbursement is typically not available for routine or preventive health care, and often begins only after a "deductible" has been satisfied, i.e. the patient has paid a certain amount of health care costs out of pocket. There may be a cap on expenses the plan will reimburse and some may be completely excluded from coverage.

As a general rule, your chances of securing coverage of BMT expenses are better if you're insured through a group plan than if you have an individual health insurance policy with the same insurance company. This is because large employers/associations can exert a great deal of influence over the private insurance company to cover extraordinary expenses, even if the basic policy does not specifically provide for payment. A 1988 survey of insurance companies by the Health Insurance Association of America found that 27 percent do not cover BMTs as a standard practice, but will do so on a case-by-case basis or at the request of an employer.

Self-Insured

A second type of insurance is the "self-insured" plan. If you're covered by a "self-insured" plan it means that your employer pays your medical claims out of company assets rather than purchasing private insurance. Benefits are outlined in a written plan description provided to plan participants. They're usually similar to benefits provided under private plans in that they allow the patient to choose his or her own doctor and hospital, do not begin reimbursing health care expenses until after a deductible has been satisfied, and may cover health care expenses only up to a certain limit.

Some employers hire a separate company (often an insurance company) to process employee insurance claims and administer payments. This arrangement can confuse people into thinking that the company hired to administer the plan is actually the insurer who defines which health care services are covered. If your employer is self-insured, the decision on benefits covered, plan limitations, and level of payment are determined by the employer, not the plan administrator.

Your chances of appealing a denial of coverage of BMT expenses are generally better if your employer is self-insured than if you're insured under a private plan or an HMO. This is because the employer is, in essence, the insurance company and therefore may have more flexibility to specify health care benefits.

HMOs (Health Maintenance Organizations)

Health maintenance organizations, or HMOs, are networks of physicians and hospitals who provide health care services to plan participants in exchange for a fixed monthly fee. Typically, there is no deductible paid by participants before coverage begins, and routine check-ups and medications often excluded from coverage under private insurance plans are usually covered. HMO participants must use the doctors/hospitals on the HMO network; they are not reimbursed for health care services provided by physicians or hospitals off the HMO network, except in extraordinary circumstances.

A common myth about HMOs is that all the procedures performed at the hospitals with which HMOs are affiliated are covered by the HMO. This is not always true. Because HMOs are very reliant on cost-containment for survival, they are sometimes more restrictive about the types of BMTs they'll cover than private insurance plans, even if BMTs are performed at a hospital on the HMO network. If approved, a patient may have little or no choice about where the BMT is to be performed.

Government Programs

Medicare is a federal program that provides health care benefits for persons 65 and older and for the disabled. The medical procedures covered by Medicare are specified in the Federal Register. Medicaid is a state-run health insurance program for persons with low incomes. Although Medicaid is funded with federal matching grants, the states largely determine the benefits provided. Some but not all BMTs are covered by Medicare and most Medicaid plans.

Comprehensive Health Insurance Plans (CHIPs) are available in several states. CHIPs provide health insurance for persons who, because of a serious health condition, cannot otherwise obtain adequate health insurance. CHIPs are typically funded by a tax on insurance companies, by state revenues, or by a combination of both. Plan participants pay an annual premium that varies according to age and sex. Most but not all CHIPs cover BMTs.

Other Plans

Blue Cross and Blue Shield plans are a type of private insurance. The "Blues" are not-for-profit organizations that negotiate fee arrangements with physicians and hospitals in a specific geographic area for health care services. Like other private plans, they offer a specific set of health care benefits in exchange for an annual premium payment. The patient pays a deductible before insurance benefits kick in, and certain medical procedures may be excluded from coverage altogether. Blue Cross/Blue Shield in some states now also offer an HMO (as do other private insurers).

Preferred Provider Organizations (PPOs) are sometimes offered as a lower cost health insurance alternative to persons covered by a group insurance plan. PPOs assemble a network of physicians, hospitals, etc. who agree to provide health care services for negotiated fees. Savings achieved through the negotiated fee arrangement are shared with plan participants via lower premiums, lower deductibles, etc.

Cancer insurance policies marketed by some companies ostensibly provide extra benefits for cancer patients. However, cancer policies often provide only minimal benefits for hospitalizations under 90 days, do not cover illness or complications arising from the cancer or treatment, and have exclusions or waiting periods that significantly reduce their value. Many experts believe they are not worth the price.

COMPREHENSIVE HEALTH INSURANCE PLANS (CHIPS)

The states below have Comprehensive Health Insurance Plans (CHIPs) for the "hard to insure."

"Yes" following a state means BMTs are not specifically excluded from coverage. However, not all BMTs or the entire cost of a BMT may be covered.

Alaska	907-349-1230	Yes
California	800-289-6574	Yes
Colorado	800-423-6174	Yes
Connecticut	800-842-0004	Yes
Florida*	904-681-9996	Yes
Illinois	800-962-8384	Yes
Indiana	800-552-7921	Yes
Iowa	800-877-5156	Yes
Kansas**	800-432-2484	Yes
Louisiana	504-926-6245	Yes
Maine	207-624-8475	Yes
Minnesota	800-382-2000 x1624	Yes
Mississippi	601-362-0799	Yes
Missouri	800-843-6447	Yes
Montana	800-447-7828	
Nebraska	800-356-3485	Yes
New Mexico	800-432-0750	Yes
North Dakota	800-737-0016	Yes
Oregon	800-542-3104	Yes
South Carolina	800-868-2503	Yes
Tennessee	800-533-9892	Yes
Utah	800-662-3398	Yes
Washington	800-877-5187	Yes
Wisconsin	800-877-1060	Yes
Wyoming	800-442-4333 x7401	

Enrollment temporarily closed
** *But the possibility of exclusion is under discussion*

IS YOUR HEALTH INSURANCE ADEQUATE?

At a minimum, your policy should provide comprehensive hospital, surgical and medical benefits including hospital room and board, anesthesia, drugs, nursing care, operating and recovery room costs, hospital lab tests, surgical procedures, doctors' fees for both office and hospital visits, and diagnostic exams and check-ups (e.g. x-rays, CAT scans, etc.).

Outpatient services (e.g. chemotherapy at the doctor's office), home

BLUE CROSS/BLUE SHIELD OPEN ENROLLMENT

The "Blues" in the states below reportedly have open enrollment periods during which persons with pre-existing medical conditions like cancer may qualify for insurance coverage. Restrictions or waiting periods may apply, and not all BMTs may be covered.

Alabama 800-292-8868
District of Columbia...............................202-484-9100
Maryland..202-484-9100
Massachusetts 800-822-2700
Michigan 800-258-8000
New Hampshire 603-228-0161
New Jersey...201-491-2729
New York 212-490-4141
North Carolina 800-222-4816
Pennsylvania 215-568-8204
Rhode Island...800-527-7290
Vermont..800-441-4094
Virginia ....202-484-9100 (DC area)
                                                           703-342-7352 (rest of state)

health care services (e.g. visiting nurses) and prescription drugs are also important benefits. If your policy requires you to pay a percentage of your medical expenses out-of-pocket, be sure there is a "stop loss clause" or maximum on medical expenses you must pay.

Check the number of days of hospitalization covered (BMTs typically require 28-56 days of hospitalization or longer), maximum benefits paid annually and over the life of the policy (BMTs typically cost $100,000 or more) and special exclusions, (e.g. whether organ transplants are covered). Be sure you're not excluded from coverage because of a pre-existing condition (such as a diagnosis of cancer prior to taking out the policy), and that there's no cancellation clause in the event your health deteriorates or you make repeated claims for coverage.

WHEN INSURANCE SAYS NO...

Don't take no for an answer. Often you can successfully challenge an insurer's refusal to pay for a BMT or other medical expenses. It will take perseverance, the cooperation of your physician, the help of your employer, and sometimes the help of an attorney, but it can be done.

There's no guarantee you'll be successful, but as a BMT patient you're already familiar with fighting tough odds!

By law, most insurers must provide you with written instructions on how to appeal a denial of coverage. Follow those instructions carefully, keeping copies of all documents sent to and received from your insurer.

If you're covered through an employee group health plan, contact your employer for help as soon as you know there's a problem. Employers can often negotiate amendments to the insurance contract or take "extra-contract" steps to cover the BMT if they're made aware of the problem early on.

What's The Problem?

To successfully challenge an insurer's refusal to pay for a BMT you must know the specific reason that coverage has been denied. By law, you're entitled to a written explanation of the denial. It may, however, be a "bare bones" explanation, requiring a follow-up letter to obtain the full details.

Insurers refuse to pre-approve or pay for BMTs for a variety of reasons. The most common are:
- the procedure is experimental or investigative
- the procedure is not medically necessary
- the patient is not eligible for benefits
- the charges exceed "usual and customary" charges for the procedure

Experimental/Investigative

BMTs are often rejected for coverage by insurers because they are "experimental" or "investigative." The definitions of experimental and investigative vary among insurers. Ask for a copy of your insurer's administrative guidelines, which spell out the circumstances under which procedures are classified as experimental or investigative.

Insurance companies may consider BMTs a covered treatment for some diseases, but experimental or investigative for others. The type of BMT proposed may also affect an insurer's determination of whether or not the procedure is experimental/investigative.

For example, an autologous BMT may be considered investigative when used to treat breast cancer, but not investigative when used to treat Hodgkin's disease. Similarly, the insurer may consider an allogeneic BMT a routine treatment for leukemia, but an autologous BMT for leukemia investigative.

The initial determination that a procedure is experimental or investigative is often made by insurance personnel with no or limited medical background. They simply apply the administrative guidelines regarding "experimental/investigative procedures" to the best of their ability, and may improperly deny coverage. It may take little more than a phone call to the insurance company medical director to reverse the denial of coverage.

Usually, however, it's not that simple. Your physician should provide the insurer with results of all studies showing the BMT to be an effective treatment for your disease, even if they're only preliminary results from on-going studies. Though the procedure is still under investigation by the medical community, there may nonetheless be sufficient evidence to persuade your insurer that a BMT provides you with the best or only chance for a cure or extended life. A 1988 survey of insurance companies by the Health Insurance Association of American found that 70 percent cover some organ transplants considered experimental/investigative.

Your physician must also convince the insurer that the BMT is a treatment option "generally accepted" by the contemporary medical community. "Generally accepted" does not mean that all physicians agree the BMT is the treatment of choice for your disease. Rather, it means that many respected experts believe it to be an effective therapy, and many physicians routinely recommend this treatment for patients. References to medical literature that cite the procedure as a therapy currently in use by the medical community as well as second opinions from other experts endorsing the use of the procedure will bolster your case.

Insurance companies sometimes rely on proclamations by Medicare, the American Medical Association, the National Institutes of Health, the U.S. Office of Technology Assessment, the American College of Physicians, the National Cancer Institute and similar groups to determine the efficacy of a medical procedure. If any of these agencies have endorsed or made positive statements regarding the use of a BMT to treat your disease, your physician should note that fact.

Your employer can play a key role in convincing the insurance company to cover your BMT. This is particularly true if your employer has had a good long-term relationship with the insurance company and/or is a large client. Employers who are self-insured have even greater flexibility to extend coverage for BMTs.

Not Medically Necessary

Most insurance policies exclude coverage of procedures that are not "medically necessary," a term whose definition can vary. Ask for a copy of the administrative guidelines relied upon by your insurer to determine the procedure is not medically necessary.

Insurers and employers often hire a "utilization review firm" (UR firm) to assess whether a procedure is medically necessary. Don't confuse the UR firm with the insurance company, or assume that a finding by the UR firm that the BMT is medically necessary means that it has been approved for payment by the insurer. A UR firm merely makes a recommendation to the insurer; that recommendation is not binding.

If coverage of a BMT or other medical expense is rejected because it's not medically necessary, your physician should prepare a letter explaining why, in your case, the procedure is medically necessary. Second opinions from other experts who've reviewed your medical records can be very helpful. Citations to medical journals and similar authorities that bolster your physician's opinion that the procedure is medically necessary will also help. If a UR firm determined that the procedure is not medically necessary, file an appeal both with the UR firm and the insurance company.

Enlist the help of your employer to persuade the insurer to reverse its initial denial of coverage. Your employer's intervention on your behalf may be very helpful, particularly if the insurance company is interested in keeping your employer happy and retaining the business.

Not Eligible

Your insurer may determine you're ineligible for coverage of BMT or other medical expenses even though they are customarily covered by the policy. This may occur if the policy contains a waiting period before coverage takes effect (e.g. you must be employed six months before being covered) or if you're excluded from coverage because of a "pre-existing condition" (i.e. you were diagnosed with the disease being treated before becoming insured by the company). Alternatively, your insurance contract may specifically exclude coverage of BMTs.

Don't despair. For all the reasons previously stated, you may be able to enlist the help of your employer to secure coverage for all or part of your BMT bills.

Usual and Customary

Even if an insurance company pre-approves payment of BMT expenses, it may subsequently refuse to pay parts of certain bills because the fees exceed "usual and customary" charges. The Health Insurance Association of America maintains a database of charges by physicians for various medical procedures, sorted by zip code. The major private insurance companies will typically pay the full cost of the procedure if it falls below the 80th or 90th percentile of charges being levied for the procedure by physicians in the same geographic area.

If part of a medical bill has been rejected because the charges exceed "usual and customary" charges, bring the problem to the attention of your physician. Sometimes, imprecise billing will cause partial denial of payment. For example, charges for two separate procedures may be lumped together under a single procedure code on the bill. When compared against the database of comparable charges for that procedure in your area, the charge will appear to be unreasonable. Have your doctor check to be sure the bill is properly itemized and the billing amount is correct before paying the balance due. If an error has been made, the bill can be resubmitted to the insurance company for payment. Otherwise, your physician may be willing to waive or reduce the charge.

DON'T TAKE "NO" FOR AN ANSWER

It is possible to get your insurance company to pay for your BMT, even if they initially deny your request. Often it will require the help of an attorney, but it can be done. Here are a few tips:

1. Don't put off meeting with the medical team at the BMT center simply because your insurer has refused to pay for the transplant. Most major BMT centers are very experienced in persuading insurers to pay for the transplant, and can help you successfully appeal an insurer's denial of coverage.
2. Don't assume the insurance company has the unilateral right to decide whether or not to cover your BMT, regardless of what language they've put in the insurance contract. Contact a lawyer to determine what your legal rights really are.
3. Don't delay in seeking the help of an attorney. Often, it takes little more than a letter from an attorney to persuade the insurance company to "rethink" its position on the issue. Usually, these types of cases can be successfully resolved for you by an attorney without actually going to court.
4. You don't know an attorney experienced with these kinds of cases in your area? Call the BMT Newsletter at 708-831-1913. We have a list of attorneys in several states who have successfully handled BMT cases. Most are also willing to talk with other attorneys who are handling these cases for the first time. If you have an attorney of your own, he or she may find the list helpful.

Going to Court

Challenging an insurance company's refusal to pay for a BMT can be difficult and time-consuming. Many BMT centers have experienced staff who can help you through the process. Nonetheless, you may be forced to sue your insurer for reimbursement of BMT bills.

Results of recently reported court cases involving patients who sued their insurer for reimbursement of BMT expenses are encouraging. Of 15 reported cases in 1990 (most involving autologous BMTs for breast cancer), preliminary injunctions or final decisions were issued in nine cases requiring insurers to pay for the BMT. Four others were resolved in the patient's favor without a trial.

The legal strategy for winning insurance reimbursement for BMTs hinges on the specific language in the insurance contract. If coverage is denied because the procedure is "experimental," "investigative" or "not generally accepted by the medical community," the court will first determine whether the contract gives the insurer the exclusive right to interpret that language in the contract. If it does not, the court will not defer to the insurer's interpretation, but will itself interpret the contract. If the contract does confer unilateral authority on the insurer to determine which procedures will be covered, the court will determine whether the insurer applied its own standards in an "arbitrary and capricious" manner. In either case, great weight is given to testimony by medical experts regarding the efficacy of the BMT in treating the disease, and whether or not the treatment is generally accepted within the medical community.

For further information on recent lawsuits involving autologous BMTs see an article by Ted Wieseman in the May 1991 issue of "Oncology Issues" published by the Journal of the Association of Community Cancer Centers.

BMT NEWSLETTER 1991 INSURANCE SURVEY

Sixty-three BMT centers from 28 states responded to the BMT Newsletter 1991 Insurance Survey. Key findings were as follows:
- 79% of the centers require insurance pre-approval before proceeding with the BMT.
- Several state-funded hospitals perform BMTs for state residents regardless of their ability to pay.
- Some private hospitals will set up special payment plans for patients when insurance will not pay for the BMT. A few have access to private funds to help patients defray BMT bills.

- 40% reported that one or more patients at their facility did not have a BMT in the last three years as a result of an insurer's refusal to pay for the procedure.
- 74% of the centers performing autologous BMTs for breast cancer reported insurance reimbursement problems.
- 44% of the centers performing autologous BMTs for ovarian cancer reported insurance reimbursement problems.
- Few centers reported reimbursement problems for autologous BMTs to treat acute leukemia, Hodgkin's disease and non-Hodgkin's lymphomas.
- 33% of the centers performing allogeneic BMTs reported reimbursement problems. Most involved an unrelated or mis-matched donor.
- Centers reported mixed results in securing reimbursement for donor-related expenses. While more than half the centers reported some reimbursement problems, even more reported at least limited success in persuading insurance to cover these costs.
- Insurance reimbursement problems were reported with all types of insurance plans—private plans, HMOs, and government programs.
- Many centers reported success in reversing an insurer's initial denial of coverage, even for therapies considered "investigative" by insurers, after intervention by the transplant physician. An initial denial of coverage by an insurer is by no means the final word.
- 38% of the centers said at least one patient had been able to raise funds privately for the BMT after being denied insurance coverage.
- 49% reported that one or more patients had sued their insurer in the past three years for coverage of their BMT expenses.

Fifty-two-year old Gail P. of Oklahoma is running on borrowed time. Diagnosed with multiple myeloma, his doctors say an autologous BMT is the only chance to prolong his life. Blue Cross/Blue Shield has refused to pay for the transplant claiming it is "experimental." He's written the following to encourage others not to give up when adversity strikes.

Because I Am A Runner, I Have A Chance
The doctor said you have multiple myeloma—CANCER.

Eight years ago I began running. I gradually built up my stamina to where I was doing six miles several times a week.

Early spring of 1990, I was looking forward to a good running season. I felt good. This would be a good year.

It started gradually, the loss of stamina, the pain in my lower back. After years of running, I was in tune with my body. I knew my body was trying to tell me something.

After numerous blood tests, the diagnosis was confirmed—multiple myeloma, an almost always fatal form of cancer that attacks the bone marrow. The doctor said I had only 27 months to live.

However, because of my running, my body was in top condition. I felt I had the strength to fight if I could find medical assistance. I found an oncologist who agreed that my body was younger than my chronological age and that I was in good physical shape. He agreed to proceed with testing and treatment. There is no question in my mind that had I not been a runner, I would not have detected the signs as early and I would not have been in good enough shape to undergo treatments.

For over 15 months I have had monthly chemotherapy and for many months shots of interferon to stimulate my immune system. No one can describe having chemotherapy to anyone else unless they have been through it.

For a while I couldn't run, couldn't even walk far. But running is such a part of me that I had to keep going to the river and hitting the path. Gradually, walking became jogging, jogging became running. I had missed our 1990 City Run, but with a good friend by my side I finished the 1991 City Run.

I may never get back to where I was before the cancer struck. But I hope to continue running and participating in my favorite races.

We're still fighting. The treatment has always been aimed at getting me to the point where a BMT could be performed. We have now reached this point. The only thing standing in the way is an insurance company that refuses to pay for the treatment.

The past months have shown me that a good positive mental attitude, strong support from my friends, and a continuous effort to run have been as important to me as all the medical treatments I have been given.

Understanding Blood Tests

Ever wonder what all those blood tests were measuring? Here's a guide to help you make sense of the results.

Complete Blood Count (CBC)

A CBC describes the number, type and form of each blood cell. It includes all tests described below.

Red Blood Cell Count (RBC)

Counts the number of red blood cells in a single drop (a microliter) of blood. "Normal" ranges vary according to age and sex.

Men: 4.5 to 6.2 million
Women: 4.2 to 5.4 million
Children: 4.6 to 4.8 million

A low RBC count may indicate anemia, excess body fluid, or hemorrhaging. A high RBC count may indicate polycythemia (an excessive number of red blood cells in the blood) or dehydration.

Total Hemoglobin Concentration

Hemoglobin gives red blood cells their color and carries oxygen from the lungs to cells. This test measures the grams of hemoglobin in a deciliter (100 ml) of blood, which can help physicians determine the severity of anemia or polycythemia. Normal values are:

Men: 14 to 18 g/dl
Women: 12 to 16 g/dl
Children: 11 to 13 g/dl

A significant anemia occurs when the hemoglobin drops below 10 g/dl.

Hematocrit

Hematocrit measures the percentage of red blood cells in the sample. Normal values vary greatly:
> **Men:** 45% to 57%
> **Women:** 37% to 47%
> **Children:** 36% to 40%

Erythrocyte (RBC) Indices

Three indices that measure the size of red blood cells and amount of hemoglobin contained in each.

Mean Corpuscular Volume (MCV) measures the volume of red blood cells. Normal is 84 to 99 fl.

Mean Corpuscular Hemoglobin (MCH) measures the amount of hemoglobin in an average cell. Normal is 26 to 32 pg .

Mean Corpuscular Hemoglobin Concentration (MCHC) measures the concentration of hemoglobin in red blood cells. Normal is 30% to 36%

White Blood Cell Count (WBC)

Measures the number of white blood cells in a drop (microliter) of blood. Normal values range from 4,100 to 10,900 but can be altered greatly by factors such as exercise, stress and disease. A low WBC may indicate viral infection or toxic reactions. A high WBC count may indicate infection, leukemia, or tissue damage. An increased risk of infection occurs once the WBC drops below 1,000/ml.

WBC Differential

Determines the percentage of each type of white blood cell in the sample. Multiplying the percentage by the total count of white blood cells indicates the actual number of each type of white blood cell in the sample. Normal values are:

Type	Percentage	Number
Neutrophil	50 - 60%	3,000 - 7,000
Eosinophils	1 - 4%	50 - 400
Basophils	0.5 - 2%	25 - 100
Lymphocytes	20 - 40%	1,000 - 4,000
Monocytes	2 - 9%	100 - 600

A serious infection can develop once the total neutrophil count (% neutrophils times total WBC) drops below 500/ml.

Platelet Count

Measures the number of platelets in a drop (microliter) of blood. Platelet counts increase during strenuous activity and in certain conditions called myeloproliferative disorders: infections, inflammations, malignancies and when the spleen has been removed. Platelet counts decrease just before menstruation. Normal values range from 150,000 to 400,000 per microliter. A count below 50,000 can result in spontaneous bleeding; below 5,000, patients are at risk of severe life-threatening bleeding.

Resources

BMT-INFORMATION/SUPPORT

BMT NEWSLETTER
1985 Spruce Ave.
Highland Park, IL 60035
708-831-1913
Bi-monthly newsletter for patients, their families and friends, and medical professionals and support organizations that work with BMT patients. Attorney referral service for patients having insurance reimbursement problems. Links prospective BMT patients with others who've been through the experience.

NATIONAL MARROW DONOR PROGRAM
3433 Broadway St. NE Ste. 400
Minneapolis, MN 55413
800-MARROW-2 800-627-7692
Offers information on becoming an unrelated volunteer bone marrow donor, and assistance to families conducting bone marrow donor drives. A patient advocate is available to answer questions and work with patients on insurance issues. Their 1995 Transplant Center Access Directory lists all BMT centers affiliated with the NMDP that perform unrelated BMT with location, diseases treated, and some cost data.

NATIONAL BMT LINK
29209 Northwestern Hwy. #624
Southfield, MI 48034
800-LINK-BMT, 800-546-5268, 810-932-8483
A national information and referral clearinghouse for BMT patients that links prospective BMT patients with BMT survivors.

BMT FAMILY SUPPORT NETWORK
P.O. Box 845
Avon, CT 06001
800-826-9376

A telephone support network for BMT patients and families.

ONCOLOGY NURSING SOCIETY
BMT Special Interest Group
501 Holiday Dr.
Pittsburgh, PA 15220-2749
412-921-7373

Publishes directory of BMT centers in the U.S. and Canada. The charge is $6 for ONS members or $7 for non-members.

AMERICAN BONE MARROW DONOR REGISTRY
Caitlin Raymond International Registry
University of Massachusetts Medical Center
55 Lake Ave. N
Worcester, MA 01655
800-726-2824

A registry of bone marrow donors; provides information on donor searches and recruitment.

BMT FUNDRAISING/FINANCIAL ASSISTANCE

ORGAN TRANSPLANT FUND
1027 S Yates
Memphis, TN 38119
800-489-3863, 901-684-1697

Helps patients in need of a BMT organize fundraisers, and maintains accounts to which tax-deductible contributions can be made on a patient's behalf.

CHILDREN'S ORGAN TRANSPLANT ASSOCIATION (COTA)
2501 Cota Dr.
Bloomington, IN 47403
800-366-2682, 812-336-8872

Helps patients in need of a BMT organize fundraisers, and maintains accounts to which tax-deductible contributions can be made on a patient's behalf.

NATIONAL CHILDREN'S CANCER SOCIETY
1015 Locust, #1040
St. Louis, MO 63101
800-532-6459

Provides financial aid to children who need a BMT, as well as fundraising advice, education, information and advocacy.

THE HLA REGISTRY FOUNDATION
70 Grand Ave.
River Edge, NJ 07661
(201)487-0883

Provides fundraising and public relations help to groups and persons organizing bone marrow donor recruitment drives.

MY FRIENDS CARE BONE MARROW TRANSPLANT FUND
(Michigan residents)
640 N. Woodward Ave., #102
Birmingham, MI 48009
810-645-5710

Provides financial assistance, support, and fundraising help for Michigan residents needing a BMT.

DEXTER JOHNSON TRUST (Oklahoma residents)
P.O. Box 26663
Oklahoma City, OK 73125
405-232-3340

Provides financial aid for children who need a BMT.

NIELSEN ORGAN TRANSPLANT FOUNDATION (Florida residents)
580 W 8th St.
Jacksonville, FL 32209
904-798-8999

Provides limited financial assistance for transplant-related expenses for residents of Nassau, Duval, St. John's, Clay and Baker counties.

THE JEFFREY KATZ FUND
4560 Fountain Ave.
Los Angeles, CA 90029
213-666-6400
Provides financial assistance to BMT patients from anywhere in the US who are transplanted at hospitals in southern California.

See also (below):
Leukemia Society of America
Leukemia Research Foundation
Children's Leukemia Foundation of Michigan
National Leukemia Association

CANCER-INFORMATION & SUPPORT

CANCER INFORMATION SERVICE
National Cancer Institute
Bldg 31 Rm 10A07
9000 Rockville Pike
Boy Scout Building, Room 340
Bethesda, MD 20892
800-422-6237
Offers a wealth of information on cancers, treatment options and clinical trials in your area.

AMERICAN CANCER SOCIETY
Attn: Patient Services Dept.
1599 Clifton Road NE
Atlanta, GA 30329
800-227-2345
Publishes brochures about various cancers and treatment options; sponsors support groups for cancer patients & their families.

CANDLELIGHTERS CHILDHOOD CANCER FOUNDATION
7910 Woodmont Ave., Ste. 460
Bethesda, MD 20814
800-366-2223
An information clearinghouse for families of children with cancer and adult survivors of childhood cancer. Publishes periodic newsletters (one for children, one for their parents) and Candlelights Guide to BMT's in Children. Sponsors parent information & support groups in many communities, and a pen-pal program for children.

NATIONAL COALITION FOR CANCER SURVIVORSHIP
1010 Wayne Ave., 5th Floor
Silver Spring, MD 20910
301-650-8868
Publishes a quarterly newsletter and advocates on behalf of cancer survivors before governmental agencies.

ANEMIA-INFORMATION AND SUPPORT

APLASTIC ANEMIA FOUNDATION OF AMERICA
P.O. Box 22689
Baltimore, MD 21203
800-747-2820
Publishes a newsletter and provides educational materials and support groups for aplastic anemia patients.

FANCONI ANEMIA RESEARCH FUND, INC.
1902 Jefferson St., Ste. 2
Eugene, OR 97405
503-687-4658
Publishes a newsletter and sponsors a support network for families of Fanconi Anemia patients.

BRAIN TUMORS-INFORMATION & SUPPORT SERVICES

NATIONAL BRAIN TUMOR FOUNDATION
785 Market St., Ste. 1600
San Francisco, CA 94103
800-934-CURE, 800-934-2873, 415-284-0208
Publishes Brain Tumors–A Guide, a periodic newsletter, and other publications of interest to persons with brain tumors. Referrals to support groups also available.

AMERICAN BRAIN TUMOR ASSOCIATION
2720 River Rd Ste. 146
Des Plaines, IL 60018
800-886-2282, 708-827-9910

Offers a Primer of Brain Tumors, a periodic newsletter, and other publications. Support group referral and a pen-pal program also available.

BREAST CANCER–INFORMATION & SUPPORT SERVICES

Y-ME NATIONAL BREAST CANCER ORGANIZATION
212 W Van Buren 4th Floor
Chicago, IL 60607
800-221-2141 weekdays 9-5
312-986-8228 24-hour hotline

Provides information on issues of interest to persons with breast cancer, a periodic newsletter, and support groups.

NATIONAL ALLIANCE OF BREAST CANCER ORGANIZATIONS
(NABCO)
9 E 37th St. 10th floor
New York, NY 10016
212-719-0154

Publishes the NABCO Breast Cancer Resource List and a quarterly newsletter available to members for a fee.

THE NEW YORK STATEWIDE BREAST CANCER HOTLINE
Adelphi University
Breast Cancer Support Program
Box 703
Garden City, NY 11530
In New York State 800-877-8077, outside 516-877-4444

Provides information about issues related to breast cancer.

LEUKEMIA, LYMPHOMAS, AND MULTIPLE MYELOMA-INFORMATION, SUPPORT & FINANCIAL ASSISTANCE

LEUKEMIA SOCIETY OF AMERICA
600 3rd Ave.
New York, NY 10016
800-955-4LSA 800-955-4572 Public Information Resource Line
212-573-8484 National Headquarters

Offers brochures, a newsletter, and videos on leukemia, myelodysplasia, lymphomas, multiple myeloma, and Hodgkins disease. Offers support groups in some areas of the country. Publishes an excellent coloring book about bone marrow transplants for children. Financial aid also available.

THE INTERNATIONAL MYELOMA FOUNDATION
2120 Stanley Hills Drive
Los Angeles, CA 90046
800-452-CURE 800-452-2873

Publishes a quarterly newsletter and provides other information on multiple myeloma at no charge. Has a hotline and offers a "patient-to-patient" network which enables patients to talk to others with multiple myeloma.

NATIONAL LEUKEMIA ASSOCIATION
585 Stewart Ave. Ste. 536
Garden City, NY 11530
516-222-1944

Provides information for leukemia patients, as well as financial assistance for drugs, x-rays, and laboratory fees.

LEUKEMIA RESEARCH FOUNDATION
(Illinois/Indiana residents within a 100-mile radius of Chicago)
4761 W. Touhy Ave., #211
Lincolnwood, IL 60646
708-982-1480

Provides financial aid, counseling, and support groups for patients with leukemia. Also conducts periodic bone marrow donor testing drives, and publishes a newsletter.

CHILDREN'S LEUKEMIA FOUNDATION OF MICHIGAN
29777 Telegraph Road Ste. 1651
Southfield, MI 48034
800-825-2536

Provides information and referral to support groups for persons with leukemia and lymphomas. Publishes a free booklet for BMT patients called Friends Helping Friends. Links prospective BMT patients with former BMT patients & their families (Michigan residents only). Some financial aid available (Michigan residents only).

IMMUNE DEFICIENCY DISORDERS

IMMUNE DEFICIENCY FOUNDATION
25 W Chesapeake Ave., Ste. 206
Towson, MD 21204
800-296-4433 410-321-6647

Publishes a quarterly newsletter. Local chapters active to varying degrees in providing patient & family support services, and educational programs.

NATIONAL ORGANIZATION FOR RARE DISORDERS (NORD)
P.O. Box 8923
New Fairfield, CT 06812-8923
800-999-NORD 800-999-6673 203-746-6518

Provides information and networking for persons with rare medical disorders.

INFERTILITY, ASSISTED REPRODUCTION, & ADOPTION

AMERICAN SOCIETY FOR REPRODUCTIVE MEDICINE
1209 Montgomery Hwy.
Birmingham, AL 35216
205-978-5000

Offers brochures on infertility and assisted reproduction.

NATIONAL ADOPTION INFORMATION CLEARINGHOUSE
5640 Nicholson Ln, Ste. 300
Rockville, MD 20852
301-231-6512

Offers a free Prospective Adoptive Parent Packet and many fact sheets, most at no charge, on support groups, single parenting, children with special needs, inter-country adoptions and home studies. Also publishes National Adoption Directory, available for $25.

NORTH AMERICAN COUNCIL ON ADOPTABLE CHILDREN (NACAC)
970 Raymond Ave., Ste. 106
St. Paul, MN 55114-1149
612-644-3036
Coalition of parent support groups for those who have adopted or are in the process of adopting special needs children.

RESOLVE INC
1310 Broadway
Somerville, MA 02144
617-623-0744 Helpline 9 am-noon, 1 pm-4 pm
Provides publications and support networks for persons struggling with infertility. Local chapters sponsor periodic seminars and support groups.

Glossary

Acute having severe symptoms and a short course.

Alkaline phosphatase an enzyme produced by the liver or bone. An elevated level of alkaline phosphatase in the blood may indicate a liver or bone problem.

ABMT autologous bone marrow transplant.

Adjuvant therapy additional drug or other treatment designed to enhance the effectiveness of the primary treatment.

Allogeneic bone marrow transplant transplant in which bone marrow from a donor, rather than the patient's own marrow, is infused.

Allograft bone marrow removed from a donor to be used in an allogeneic BMT.

Alopecia loss of hair.

Anemia too few red blood cells in the bloodstream, resulting in insufficient oxygen to tissues and organs.

Anaphalaxis acute allergic reaction shortness of breath, rash, wheezing, hypotension.

Antibiotic a drug used to fight bacterial infections.

Antibody a protein produced by the body, in response to a foreign substance, that fights the invading organism.

Antiemetic a drug used to control nausea and vomiting.

Antigen a substance that evokes a response from the body's immune system resulting in the production of antibodies or other defensive action by white blood cells.

Apheresis a painless procedure by which blood is withdrawn from a patient's arm and circulated through a machine that removes certain components and returns the remaining components to the patient. This procedure is used to remove platelets from platelet donors' blood, or stem cells from patients undergoing a peripheral stem cell harvest.

Aplasia a failure to develop or form. In bone marrow "aplasia," the marrow cavity is empty.

Ascites accumulation of fluid in the stomach area.

Ataxia loss of balance.

Autologous bone marrow transplant transplant in which the patient's own bone marrow, rather than marrow from a donor, is infused during transplant to provide the body with a source of stem cells.

Autograft bone marrow removed from the patient to be used in an autologous BMT.

Bacteria microscopic organisms that invade human cells, multiply rapidly, and produce toxins that interfere with normal cell functions.

Baseline test test which measures an organ's normal level of functioning. Used to determine if any changes in organ function occur following treatment.

Bilirubin a pigment produced when the liver processes waste products. A high bilirubin level causes yellowing of the skin.

Biopsy removal of tissue for examination under a microscope, sometimes required to enable the doctor to make a proper diagnosis.

Blast cell immature cell.

Blast crisis in patients with chronic myelogenous leukemia, the progression of the diseases to an "acute" advanced phase, evidenced by an increased number of immature white blood cells in the circulating blood. Sometimes loosely used to describe a rapid increase in the white blood cell count of any leukemic patient.

Bone marrow spongy tissue in the cavities of large bones, where the body's blood cells are produced.

Bone marrow aspiration procedure used to remove a sample of bone marrow, usually from the rear hip bone, for examination under the microscope.

Cardiac pertaining to the heart.

Catheter small, flexible plastic tube inserted into a portion of the body to administer or remove fluids.

CBC complete blood count. Determines whether the proper number of red blood cells, white blood cells and platelets are present in the patient's blood.

Central line see central venous catheter.

Central venous catheter small, flexible plastic tube inserted into the large vein above the heart, through which drugs and blood products can be given, and blood samples withdrawn painlessly (also called central line; Hickman catheter).

Chemo-responsive responds to chemotherapy, e.g., a tumor is chemo-responsive if it shrinks in size following chemotherapy.

Chemotherapy drug or combination of drugs designed to kill cancerous cells.

Chronic persisting for a long time.

Clinical trial a study of the effectiveness of a drug or treatment.

CMV see cytomegalovirus.

CNS central nervous system.

Colony stimulating factor proteins that stimulate the production and growth of certain types of blood cells.

Conditioning see preparative regimen.

Conjunctivitis eye inflammation.

Contracture shortening of muscle, skin and other soft tissue, usually in the limbs. May occur in patients with chronic graft-versus-host disease.

Cryopreservation to preserve by freezing. Bone marrow harvested for an autologous BMT, for example, is cryopreserved.

CSF see colony stimulating factor.

CT-scan also called a CAT-scan or CT-X-ray. A three-dimensional x-ray.

Cytomegalovirus a virus that lies dormant in many persons' bodies and frequently causes infection post-transplant. Patients who have been exposed to and still carry the virus are CMV-positive.

Dermatitis a skin rash.

Dysplasia alteration in the size, shape and organization of cells or tissues.

-ectomy surgical removal.

Edema abnormal accumulation of fluid, e.g., pulmonary edema refers to a build-up of fluid in the lungs.

EKG (Electrocardiogram) test to determine the pattern of a patient's heartbeat.

Electrolyte minerals found in the blood such as sodium potassium that must be maintained within a certain range to prevent organ malfunction.

-emia of the blood; usually refers to a blood disorder, e.g., leukemia or anemia

Emesis vomit.

Encephalopathy abnormal functioning of the brain.

Engraftment when bone marrow infused during a BMT "takes" or is accepted by the patient, and begins producing blood cells.

Enzyme a protein that is capable of facilitating a chemical reaction.

Eosinophil a type of white blood cell that protects against infection.

Febrile feverish.

Foley catheter flexible plastic tube inserted into the bladder to provide continuous urinary drainage.

Fungus a primitive life form that can cause infection in the body. Fungi that sometimes cause post-transplant infections are the Candida and Aspergillus fungi.

Gastritis inflammation of the stomach.

Gastrointestinal refers to the stomach and intestines.

G-CSF granulocyte colony stimulating factor. A protein that stimulates the growth and maturation of granulocytes.

GM-CSF granulocyte-macrophage colony stimulating factor. A protein that stimulates the growth and maturation of a wide variety of white blood cells.

Graft rejection when donated bone marrow infused during a BMT is rejected by the patient's body or doesn't "take."

Graft-versus-host disease a condition that can occur following an allogeneic BMT in which some of the donor's bone marrow cells attack the patient's tissues and organs.

Granulocyte a sub-class of white blood cells, so named because of the presence of granules in the cell. These cells protect the body against bacterial infections.

Growth factor see colony stimulating factor.

GVHD see graft-versus-host disease.

Hematocrit the percentage of the blood made up of red blood cells.

Hematology the study of blood and its disorders.

Hemoglobin the part of red blood cells that carries oxygen to tissues.

Hemorrhage bleeding.

Hemorrhagic cystitis bladder ulcers.

Hepat(o)- pertaining to the liver.

Hepatitis inflammation of the liver.

Hickman catheter see central venous line.

HLA see human leukocyte antigen.

Human leukocyte antigen a genetic "fingerprint" on white blood cells and platelets, composed of proteins that play a critical role in activating the body's immune system to respond to foreign organisms.

Hyper- excessive, increased.

Hyperalimentation intravenous feeding that provides patients with all essential nutrients when they're unable to feed themselves. Also called hyperal, TPN or total parenteral nutrition.

Hyperpigmentation darkening of the skin.

Hypertension high blood pressure.

Hypo- a deficiency, less than usual.

Hypotension low blood pressure.

Iliac crest the hip bone in which a large quantity of bone marrow is concentrated.

Immune system the body's defense network against infection and foreign particles.

Immunocompromised a condition in which the immune system is not functioning normally.

Immunoglobulin an antibody.

Immunosuppression a condition in which the patient's immune system is functioning at a lower than normal level. Allogeneic BMT patients are deliberately immunosuppressed to allow the donor's bone marrow to engraft without interference from the patient's immune system.

-itis inflammation.

Intravenous through a vein.

Jaundice yellowing of the skin and eyes. A sign that the liver is not functioning properly.

Karnofsky score a measure of the patient's overall physical health following a BMT, judged by his or her level of activity.

Laminar air flow unit an air-filtering system used at some transplant facilities to remove particulate matter and fungi from the air.

Leukocyte white blood cell.

Lymphocyte a type of white blood cell that helps protect the body against invading organisms by producing antibodies and regulating the immune system response.

Macrophage a type of white blood cell that assists in the body's fight against bacteria and infection by engulfing and destroying invading organisms.

Malabsorption failure of intestines to properly absorb oral medications or nutrients from food.

Mentation thinking.

Metabolite a by-product of the breakdown of either food or medication by the body.

Metastatic spread of a disease from the organ or tissue of origin to another part of the body.

Mixed lymphocyte culture test to determine whether a patient's and donor's white blood cells interact adversely. Often used to determine whether a person would be a suitable bone marrow donor for a particular patient.

MLC mixed lymphocyte culture.

Monoclonal antibody antibodies that are all identical, derived from a single "clone." Sometimes used in "purging," a process by which certain cells are removed from bone marrow before infusion into patients.

Monocyte a type of white blood cell that assists in the fight against bacteria and fungi that invade the body.

Morbidity sickness; side effects and symptoms of a treatment or disease.

MRI magnetic resonance imaging. A method of taking pictures of body tissue using magnetic fields and radio waves.

Mucositis mouth sores.

Neuro- pertaining to the nervous system.

Neutropenia a deficiency of neutrophils.

Neutrophil a type of white blood cell that is the body's primary defense against harmful bacteria.

NPO do not take anything by mouth.

Oncology the study of cancer.

Oto- pertaining to the ear.

Packed red blood cells red blood cells collected from one individual that are packed into a small volume for transfusion into a patient.

Palliative provides relief.

Pancytopenia a deficiency of all types of blood cells.

-pathy disease.

-penia deficiency, e.g., neutropenia means a deficiency of a type of white blood cell called a neutrophil.

Peripheral neuropathy injury to the nerves that supply sensation to the arms and legs.

Petechiae small red spots on the skin that usually indicate a low platelet count.

Phlebitis inflammation of a vein.

-plasia development, formation

Plasma the fluid and protein-containing portion of the blood.

Platelets the smallest cell elements in the blood, needed to control bleeding.

Polycythemia an increase in the total number of red blood cells in the bloodstream.

Preparative regimen the chemotherapy and/or radiation given to BMT patients prior to transplant to kill diseased cells and/or make space for healthy new marrow and/or suppress the immune system so graft rejection does not occur.

Prognosis the predicted or likely outcome.

Prophylactic preventive measure or medication.

Protocol the plan of treatment.

Pulmonary pertaining to the lungs

Purging process by which certain types of cells are removed from bone marrow prior to infusion into the BMT patient. In autologous BMTs, marrow may be purged to remove lingering cancerous cells. In allogeneic BMTs, donor bone marrow may be purged to remove cells that cause graft-versus-host disease.

RBC red blood cell.

Red blood cell cells that pick up oxygen from the lungs and transport it to tissues throughout the body.

Relapse recurrence of the disease following treatment.

Remission, complete condition in which no cancerous cells can be detected by a microscope, and the patient appears to be disease-free.

Remission, partial generally means that by all methods used to measure the existence of a tumor, there has been at least a 50 percent regression of the disease following treatment.

Renal pertaining to the kidney.

Sepsis the presence of organisms in the blood.

SGOT an enzyme produced by the liver. Elevated levels of SGOT in the blood indicate a liver problem.

SGPT an enzyme produced by the liver. Elevated levels of SGPT in the blood indicate a liver problem.

Solid tumor a cancer that originates in organ or tissue other than bone marrow or the lymph system.

Stem cell "mother" blood cells from which several different types of blood cells evolve.

Steroid in bone marrow transplantation, a drug commonly used in combination with other drugs to prevent and control graft-versus-host disease.

Stomatitis mouth sores.

Subclavian catheter see central venous catheter.

Syngeneic bone marrow transplant transplant in which an identical twin is the bone marrow donor.

T-cell a type of white blood cell that can distinguish which cells belong in a person's body and which do not.

TBI total body irradiation.

Thrombocyte see platelet

Total parenteral nutrition intravenous feeding that provides patients with all essential nutrients when they're unable to feed themselves. Also called TPN, hyperalimentation or hyperal.

Toxin poison.

TPN see total parenteral nutrition.

Trauma injury.

Tumor uncontrolled growth of abnormal cells in an organ or tissue.

Tumor burden the size of the tumor or number of abnormal cells in the organ or tissue.

Ultrasound a technique for taking a picture of internal organs or other structures using sound waves.

Veno-occlusive disease a disease that sometimes occurs following high-dose chemotherapy and/or radiation, in which the blood vessels that carry blood through the liver become swollen and clogged.

Virus a tiny parasite-like agent that invades organisms, such as human cells, and alters their genetic machinery, turning them into factories for production of more of the virus.

VOD see veno-occlusive disease.

WBC white blood cell count.

Whole blood blood that has not been separated into its various components.

Xerostomia dryness of the mouth caused by malfunctioning salivary glands.

Index

ABMT (see bone marrow transplant, autologous)
Actigall 107
acute graft-versus-host disease (see graft-versus-host disease, acute)
acute granulocytic leukemia (see also acute myelogenous leukemia) 38
acute GVHD (see graft-versus-host disease, acute)
acute lymphocytic leukemia 27-28, 39, 47
acute megakaryocytic leukemia (see also acute myelogenous leukemia) 38
acute monocytic leukemia (see also acute myelogenous leukemia) 38
acute myelogenous leukemia..27-28, 38-39, 47, 134
acute nonlymphocytic leukemia (see also acute myelogenous leukemia).27-28, 38, 47
acute promyelocytic leukemia (see also acute myelogenous leukemia) 38
acyclovir 86-88
adenovirus 88-89, 106
adoption 63, 69, 109, 119-121, 149-150
Adriamycin...112, 113
AFS (see American Fertility Society)
AIDS testing 115
air filtering equipment..17, 85, 155
alkaline phosphatase 102, 104, 105, 107, 151
alkylating agents..112
ALL (see acute lymphocytic leukemia)
allogeneic bone marrow transplant (see bone marrow transplant, allogeneic)
alopecia (see hair loss)
American Bone Marrow Donor Registry 33
American Fertility Society...118, 149
aminoglycosides..84
AML (see acute myelogenous leukemia)
amphotericin B 85, 86, 105
anemia...137, 151, 153
anesthesia 13, 14, 43, 49, 116, 127
anger 17, 55, 57, 68, 97, 98
ANLL (see acute nonlymphocytic leukemia)
anti-depressant medication 59
anti-fungal medication 85
anti-nausea medication 15
anti-viral medication 86, 87
antibiotics 16, 84, 85, 96, 104-105, 151

antibody 21, 30, 81, 82, 83-84, 86, 151, 154, 155
antigen 34-37, 40, 41, 42, 82-83, 151, 154
antithymocyte globulin..40
apheresis 48, 151
aplastic anemia 11, 33, 38, 40-42, 53, 67-68, 99, 103, 113, 145
appetite, loss of...107
ara-C (see also cytosine arabinoside, cytarabine) 112-113
artificial insemination 109, 114-116, 118
ascites (see also fluid accumulation) 103, 151
Aspergillus...85-86, 153
assisted reproduction (see medically assisted reproduction)
Association of American Cancer Centers..133
ATG (see antithymocyte globulin)..40
autologous bone marrow transplant (see bone marrow transplant, autologous)
autologous stem cell transplant (see peripheral stem cell transplant)
autotransplant (see bone marrow transplant, autologous)
azathioprine 107
B-cell..21, 22, 23, 82, 83, 86
bacteria...........................16, 17, 18, 21, 35, 81, 82, 83-84, 85, 90, 93, 105, 152, 155
bactrim 90, 96
baseline tests..13
basophil 21, 22, 47, 138
BCNU (see carmustine)
bile...101, 102, 104, 105, 106, 107
bile duct 101, 102, 104, 106
biliary disease 8, 106
biliary sludge 106
bilirubin...101, 102, 104, 105, 107, 152
bladder 84, 111, 112, 153, 154
blast cell...152
bleeding 16, 17, 22, 26, 27, 31, 40, 89, 139, 154, 156
blood pressure, low 83, 154
blood transfusion 16, 17, 18, 41, 77, 106, 156
blood tests...12, 43, 102, 135, 137-139
Blue Cross...50, 126, 128, 134
Blue Shield 50, 126, 128, 134
BMT Newsletter...49, 69, 123, 132-133, 141, 148
bone marrow
    aspirate..58
    cryopreservation 14, 49, 114, 153
    definition 11-13, 154
    donor..11, 12, 25, 33-34, 37, 40-44, 73, 87, 123, 141
    engraftment (see engraftment)
    harvest... 13-14, 43, 49
    purging..13, 14, 28, 30-31, 38, 104, 155, 156
    T-cell depletion (see bone marrow, purging)
bone marrow donor
    matched related 12, 33-34, 36-40, 91
    mismatched..33, 37, 40-41, 91, 96, 103, 104, 123, 133
    unrelated 33, 37, 41-42, 91, 96, 103, 104, 133

bone marrow rescue (see bone marrow transplant, autologous)
bone marrow transplant
    allogeneic..12, 25, 29, 33-45, 81, 85, 87, 88, 89,
                                            91, 93, 97, 104, 107, 151, 154
    autologous....................................12, 14, 25-33, 38, 39, 42, 47, 49, 50, 81, 85, 87,
                                  88, 92, 123, 129, 133, 134, 151, 152, 153
        hospitalization period..13-18
        mis-matched related donor.......................33, 37, 40-41, 91, 96, 103, 104, 123, 133
        mis-matched unrelated donor...42
        pediatric..25, 29, 67-79
        pre-transplant tests...13
        quality of life after..18-19
        syngeneic...12, 25, 107, 157
        unrelated donor...37, 41-42, 91, 96, 103, 104, 133
brain tumor...13, 30, 47, 48, 113, 146
breast cancer.................11, 12, 23, 25, 28-29, 31-32, 47, 48, 50, 113, 123, 129, 133, 134, 146
bronchitis..83, 96
busulfan...112, 113
cancer insurance...126
Candida..85-86, 105, 153
carmustine..112
CT scan..102, 153
CBC (complete blood count)...137, 152
cDDP (see also cisplatin)..112
cell lysis..83
cell separation machine..48
central line (see central venous line)
central venous line (see also Hickman catheter)..15, 154
cephalosporin...84
cervix...112
CGL (see chronic granulocytic leukemia)
chemo-responsive..152
chemotherapy.....12, 14, 15, 23, 26, 27, 28, 29, 31, 34, 38, 39, 41, 49, 50, 58, 63, 69, 81, 83,
                     86, 102, 103, 109, 112-114, 116, 117, 127, 135, 152, 156, 157
        consolidation...38
        induction..38
chicken pox..81, 88-89
children...28, 29, 38, 39, 40, 42, 67-79, 109,
                    114, 116, 119-121, 142-144, 147, 150
chills..15
CHIPs (comprehensive health insurance plans)...126-127
chlorambucil..112, 113
chronic graft-versus-host disease (see graft-versus-host disease, chronic)
chronic GVHD (see graft-versus-host disease, chronic)
chronic granulocytic leukemia (see chronic myelogenous leukemia)
chronic myelogenous leukemia...27, 39, 44, 95, 152
cisplatin..112, 113
CML (see chronic myelogenous leukemia)
CMV (see cytomegalovirus)
CMV pneumonia (see cytomegalovirus)
colony stimulating factor...21, 23, 48, 153-154

Comfort, Georgia 32
committed progenitor cell..23, 48
complement 22, 30, 83
complete blood count...137, 152
comprehensive health insurance plan..126-127
conditioning (see preparative regimen)
confusion 17, 94, 97, 102-103
consolidation chemotherapy (see chemotherapy, consolidation)
contractures...95, 96, 97
corpus luteum 111
cramping...48, 93
cryopreservation
    bone marrow 14, 49, 114, 153
    embryo..63, 115, 118
    sperm...114
CT X-ray (see CT-scan)
cyclophosphamide...92, 112, 113
cyclosporine...40, 45, 94, 96, 104, 107
cytarabine (see also ara-C)...112
cytomegalovirus 85-87, 106, 152-153
cytosine arabinoside (see also ara-C)...112
Cytoxan (see also cyclophosphamide)...112-113
D., Thelda 50
depression 60, 68, 71, 73, 97
dialysis 103
diarrhea...16, 93, 97
diuretic 103
DNA typing 37
drug dependency 59
donor oocyte (see oocyte, donor)
donor sperm (see sperm, donor)
doxorubicin 112
DTIC 112
EBV (see Epstein-Barr virus)
edema (see also swelling)...103, 153
embryo...109, 110, 111, 112, 114, 116, 117
    donation 109, 116-118
    preservation (see cryopreservation, embryo)
emotional stress (see also stress) 17
emotional support..55, 56, 59-61, 62, 98, 142, 144-148, 150
endometrium 110
engraftment 15, 16, 41, 94, 153
    delayed 30
eosinophil...21, 22, 47, 138, 153
epididymis...111
Epstein-Barr virus...88, 89, 106
erythrocyte (see also red blood cell) 11, 21, 47
erythrocyte indices..138
erythroleukemia...38
estrogen 110, 111, 116
Ewing's sarcoma 30

eye problems 87, 88, 90, 93, 97, 153
face mask...16, 17, 61, 63, 89
fallopian tube 110-111, 114
Fanconi's anemia...145
feeding, intravenous...105, 154, 157
fertilization...109-112, 114, 116-118
fetus...110
fever 15, 16, 21, 86, 89, 103, 105, 106
fimbria...111
fluconazole 86, 105
fluid accumulation...102, 103
follicle...110, 111
follicle stimulating hormone 110, 111, 116
FSH (see follicle stimulating hormone)
fungus 16, 21, 81, 84, 85-86, 90, 93, 101, 104, 105, 107, 153, 155
    Aspergillus 85-86, 153
    Candida...85-86, 105, 153
G-CSF...48
gallbladder 101, 106
gallstones 102, 106
gamete intrafallopian tube transfer 117
ganciclovir...86, 88
gastrointestinal tract 27, 89
genetic disease 38
GIFT 78, 117
GM-CSF 48, 154
graft rejection 12, 37, 41, 92-93, 154, 156
graft-versus-host disease...........................12, 14, 16, 17, 25, 34, 35, 37, 40, 41, 42, 45, 63,
    69, 81, 85, 86, 88, 91-99, 104, 105, 106, 107, 153, 154, 156, 157
    acute 91, 92-95, 104, 106, 107
    anti-leukemic effect...94-95
    chronic 45, 91, 94, 95-97, 104, 107, 153
    coping with the stress...97-99
graft-versus-leukemia (see graft-versus-host disease, anti-leukemic effect)
Graham-Pole MD, John...65
granulocyte...21, 31, 105, 107, 153, 154
granulocyte-colony stimulating factor...48
granulocyte-macrophage colony stimulating factor 48
growth factor...48, 154
GVHD (see graft-versus-host disease)
HCG (see human chorionic gonadotropin)
hair
    loss 54, 58, 61, 95-96
    facial...94
    premature graying 95-96
haplotype 36-37, 42
harvest (see bone marrow harvest, peripheral stem cell harvest)
HDC (see chemotherapy, high-dose)
heart...13, 83, 103, 152
helplessness 17-18, 57
Health Insurance Association of America...124, 130-131, 149

health maintenance organization...125
hematocrit..138, 154
hemoglobin 137, 138, 154
hemorrhaging (see also bleeding)...137
hepatic artery 101
hepatitis..101, 103, 106, 107, 154
hepatocytes...101
herpes simplex virus..85, 86-87, 106
Hickman catheter...15, 84, 152, 154
high-dose chemotherapy (see chemotherapy, high-dose)
HIAA 124, 130-131, 149
HIV..115
hives..15, 21
HLA (see human leukocyte antigen system)
    loci..35
    matching 37
    typing...34, 37, 92
HMO (see health maintenance organization)
Hodgkin's disease.....................11, 25, 27, 30, 33, 39, 47, 48, 68, 109, 112, 113, 129, 134
human chorionic gonadotropin...111, 116
human leukocyte antigen system 34-37, 42, 92, 154
human menopausal gonadatropin 116
human papilloma virus 89
HPV (see human papilloma virus)
HSV (see herpes simplex virus)
hydroxyurea..39
hyperalimentation (see feeding, intravenous)
ifosfamide 112, 113
iliac crest 13, 154
immune deficiency diseases........................11, 33, 38, 40,42, 67, 103, 148
immune system................................11, 16, 21, 35, 57, 81-84, 90, 92, 93, 96,
                                                                              105, 107, 111, 154
immuncompromised...81, 154
immunoglobulin...21, 87, 88, 154
immunosuppression 92, 94, 154
immunotoxins...30
Imuran...107
in-vitro fertilization..116-119
inborn errors of metabolism..67
induction chemotherapy (see chemotherapy, induction)
infection...11, 16, 17, 19, 21, 25, 26, 27, 31, 40, 57,
...................................81-90, 93, 96, 99, 101, 103, 104-105, 106, 107, 138, 139, 151, 153, 154
    bacterial (see also bacteria)...21, 83-84, 85, 96
    bladder...84
    bloodstream 104
    brain 87, 90
    ear 83
    eyes...97, 88, 90
    fungal..85-86, 104-105
    genital..86
    intestines 84, 85, 87, 89, 105

kidneys..89, 105
liver...17, 87, 90, 104, 105, 106, 107
lungs...84, 85, 87, 89, 90
lymph system 89
mouth...84, 85, 86, 87
muscles..90
prevention...84, 85, 87, 88, 89, 90
protozoa 21, 90
rectum 86
sinus 83, 85
skin 84, 87, 88
spleen 105
viral..21, 85, 86-89, 99, 106, 138
infertility 63, 69, 70, 109-121, 149
interferon 39, 107, 135
interleukins...23
International Bone Marrow Transplant Registry 38
intestines 84, 85, 87, 89, 93, 95, 101, 105, 106, 107, 153, 155
isolation...17, 57, 61
insurance...43, 115, 117, 121, 123-135, 141, 148-149
   cancer 126
   BMT Newsletter 1991 Survey 133-134
   exclusion of coverage 128-132
irradiation, total body 12, 14, 15, 23, 26, 27, 28, 29, 31, 32, 34, 41, 49, 50,
     58, 63, 81, 83, 86, 92, 102, 103, 109, 112, 113-114, 116, 117, 156, 157
IVF Registry...117
IVF (see in vitro fertilization)
jaundice..93, 95, 96, 98, 102, 103, 104, 105, 107, 155
kidney...13, 89, 94, 102, 103, 105, 156
l-Pam...112, 113
LAF (see laminar air flow)
laminar air flow (see air filtering equipment)
laparoscopy 116
leukemia..11, 23, 25, 26, 27-28, 30, 33, 38-39, 41, 42,
     44, 47, 48, 53, 67-68, 95, 103, 109, 113, 129, 134, 138, 143, 147-148
leukocyte (see also neutrophil, granulocytes, eosinophils, basophils, monocytes,
   lymphocytes, T-cells, B-cells)....................................11, 21, 34, 82-83, 92, 154, 155
leuprolide..116
LH (see luteinizing hormone)
liver 17, 45, 54, 87, 90, 93, 95-97, 99, 101-107, 151, 152, 154, 155, 157
   biopsy..102
   enzymes...102, 105, 157
   hepatic artery...101
   hepatocytes 101
   infection (see infection, liver)
   portal vein 101
   problems following GVHD...17, 93, 99, 104, 105
   swelling and tenderness..102
lungs..21, 83, 84, 85, 87, 89, 90, 95, 96, 103, 137, 153, 156
   infection (see infection, lungs; also cytomegalovirus)
Lupron...116

luteinizing hormone..111
lymph nodes..27
lymph system 82, 89, 157
lymphocytes (see also T-cells, B-cells) 21-22, 23, 27, 37, 47, 82, 104, 138, 155
lymphoid stem cell...22-23
lymphoma 11, 12, 13, 25, 26-27, 30, 33, 38, 39, 47, 48, 51, 103, 113, 134, 147
        Hodgkin's disease.................11, 12, 25, 26-27, 30, 33, 39, 47, 48, 112, 113, 134, 147
        non-Hodgkin's...............................11, 13, 25, 26-27, 30, 33, 47, 48, 51, 113, 134, 147
macrophage 21, 22, 82, 83, 155
malabsorption (see stomach disorders)
MCH (see mean corpuscular hemoglobin)
MCHC (see mean corpuscular hemoglobin concentration)
MCV (see mean corpuscular volume)
mean corpuscular hemoglobin...138
mean corpuscular hemoglobin concentration.....................................138
mean corpuscular volume...138
mechlorethamine hydrochloride...112
Medicaid...126, 143
medically assisted reproduction 69, 109, 114-119
Medicare...126, 130
megakaryocyte...22
melphalan 112
metabolic storage diseases...38
methotrexate 94, 104
Metrodin 116
mis-matched bone marrow (see bone marrow donor, mismatched)
mismatched bone marrow transplant (see bone marrow transplant, mismatched)
Mitchell, Susan...99
mixed lymphocyte culture test 155
MLC (see mixed lymphocyte culture test)
monoclonal antibodies..30, 155
monocyte...21, 22, 47, 82, 83, 138, 155
mood swings 94, 97-98
MOPP 113
mouth
        cleaning and care during BMT..84, 95
        dryness..96, 157
        infection..84, 85, 86, 87
        problems following GVHD...95
        sores..17, 45, 54, 58, 87, 96, 155, 157
mucositis (see mouth, sores)
multiple myeloma...............................11, 33, 47, 48, 113, 134-135, 147
muscle, infection..90
myelodysplasia...33
myelodysplastic syndrome (see myelodysplasia)
myeloid stem cell..22-23
myeloproliferative disorder 139
Myleran (see busulfan)
National Marrow Donor Program.......................................33, 42-43, 141, 149
natural killer cells 83
nausea 16, 93, 105, 151

neuroblastoma 25, 29, 30, 47, 48, 67
neurological problems..94
neutropenia...84, 155, 156
neutrophil.......................................21, 22, 47, 82, 83, 84, 138-139, 155
nitrogen mustard...112, 113
NMDP (see National Marrow Donor Program)
non-Hodgkin's lymphoma (see lymphoma)
oocytes..110
oocyte, donor 116-118
Oncology Issues 133
oral hygiene (see mouth, cleaning and care)
osteopetrosis..34
ovarian cancer 11, 12, 23, 25, 30, 47, 48, 113, 134
ovary 110, 111
pain 14, 17, 54, 58-59, 76, 88, 95, 96, 103, 105, 106
pancreas, inflammation of..106
papovavirus 88
parasites 21
pediatric bone marrow transplant...67-79
penicillin 84, 96
pergonal 116
peripheral blood...48, 49, 50
peripheral stem cell harvest/transplant 47-51, 151
phagocytes...83
P., Gail...134
plasma 156
platelet................11, 16, 22, 23, 31, 40, 44, 45, 47, 48, 51, 60, 139, 151, 152, 154, 156, 157
pluripotent stem cell..22-23, 47
Pneumocystis Carinii 90
pneumonia..84, 85, 87, 88, 89, 90, 96
polycythemia 156
PPO (see Preferred Provider Organization)
precursor cell..23
Preferred Provider Organization 126
preleukemia (see myelodysplasia)
prednisone 96, 104, 105, 107, 113
pregnancy..109-111, 114-119
preparative regimen...14, 41, 103, 153, 156
procarbazine..112, 113
progesterone...111, 116
prostate gland 112
protocol..14, 156
protozoa...21, 90
PSCH (see peripheral stem cell harvest)
psychiatric help 59
psychological stress (see also stress)..17
psychological support (see also support group, support person).................13
puberty...70
purging, bone marrow...................................13, 14, 28, 30-31, 38, 156
radiation (see irradiation)
RBC (see red blood cell count)

RBC indices 138
red blood cell......................11, 16, 21, 22, 23, 40, 48, 101, 103, 137, 138, 151, 152, 154, 156
    count 137, 138, 156
Reed-Sternberg cell 27
relapse 19, 28, 29, 30, 38, 39, 69, 94, 95, 119, 156
remission..12, 27, 28, 29, 38-39, 156
reproductive cells 109, 112, 113
reproductive organ...113
resentment 17, 68
respiratory syncitial virus..89
RSV (see respiratory syncitial virus)
sarcoma 30, 48
SART (see Society for Assisted Reproductive Technology)
sedative 57
seizures...94
self-insurance...124, 125, 130
semen 112, 115
seminal vesicles...110, 111
seminiferous tubule..110, 111
Septra..90
sexual intercourse 87, 111, 112
SGOT...102, 105, 157
SGPT...102, 105, 157
shingles...88
shock...83
siblings 12, 33, 34, 37, 40, 41, 68, 70, 71, 72-73, 77, 78, 95, 120
sinusoid 101
skin
    blistering..88, 93
    discoloration 95, 96
    lesions..87
    peeling..93
    tautness..95, 96
    rash...45, 88, 93, 95, 96, 153
small cell lung cancer 47, 113
Society for Assisted Reproductive Technology 118
solid tumor...30, 67, 103, 157
sperm banking 63, 69, 109, 114-115
sperm donation...109, 115
spermatid 111
spermatocyte 111
spleen 22, 27, 105, 139
stem cell 11, 12, 22-23, 47-48, 49, 50, 51, 82, 151, 152, 157
    lymphoid...22
    myeloid..22
    pluripotent 22, 47
steroid...40, 157
stomach disorders 93, 95, 96, 97, 151, 153
stress 17, 53, 56-64, 74, 77, 97-98, 109, 138
support group...56, 146, 148
support person 60-62

swelling...102, 103, 153
syngeneic bone marrow transplant (see bone marrow transplant, syngeneic)
T-cell......................14, 21, 22, 23, 35, 40, 41, 82-83, 86, 90, 91-92, 93, 94-95, 104, 157
    CD-8...95
    depletion (see bone marrow, purging)
    helper...82
    killer..82
    purging (see bone marrow, purging)
    suppressor...82
taste, altered...58
TBI (see irradiation, total body irradiation)
testicles..111
testicular cancer...25, 30, 47, 48, 113
thalassemia..33, 38
thalidomide..96
thinking, confused or changed (see confusion)
thiotepa...112, 113
thrombocyte (see also platelet)...157
thymus gland...22, 35
tissue typing..34, 92
total body irradiation (see irradiation, total body)
total hemoglobin concentration...137
toxin..83, 101, 102, 103, 152, 157
Toxoplasma Gondii...90
toxoplasmosis..90
TPN (see feeding, intravenous)
transfusion (see blood transfusion)
tumor..23, 26, 27, 29, 30, 67, 83, 146, 152, 156, 157
unrelated bone marrow donor (see bone marrow donor, unrelated)
unrelated donor bone marrow transplants (see bone marrow transplant, unrelated donor)
ultrasound guided needle aspiration...116
urethra...110, 112
urine...89
urologic cancer..113
ursodeoxycholic acid..107
uterus..110, 111, 112, 114, 115, 116, 117
utilization review firm...131
vaccinations...89, 96
vagina..85, 110, 111, 112, 114
vancomycin..84
varicella zoster virus..85, 88, 106
Velban...112, 113
veno-occlusive disease..102-103, 157
vinblastine..112

virus 16-17, 85, 86-89, 102, 106, 107, 115, 153, 157
    adenovirus 88, 106
    cytomegalovirus 85, 86, 87-88, 106, 152, 153
    echovirus 106
    Epstein-Barr...88, 89, 106
    hepatitis B...106
    hepatitis C 107
    herpes simplex..85, 86-87, 106
    human papilloma 89
    papovavirus...88
    respiratory syncitial..89
    varicella zoster 85, 86, 88, 106
VOD (see veno-occlusive disease)
VZV (see virus, varicella zoster)
WBC differential...138
weight gain 94, 98, 102, 103
weight loss...95, 96
white blood cell (see also leukocyte)..........11, 16, 18, 21, 23, 27, 34-35, 39, 40, 41, 47, 48,
                81, 82-83, 84, 91, 104, 105, 107, 138, 151, 152, 153, 154, 155, 156, 157
    count 39, 107, 138, 152, 157
Wise, Laura...44
xerostomia (see mouth, dryness)
ZIFT (see zygote intrafallopian tube transfer)
zygote intrafallopian tube transfer..117